BY RICHARD SELZER

MORTAL LESSONS: NOTES ON THE ART OF SURGERY
LETTERS TO A YOUNG DOCTOR

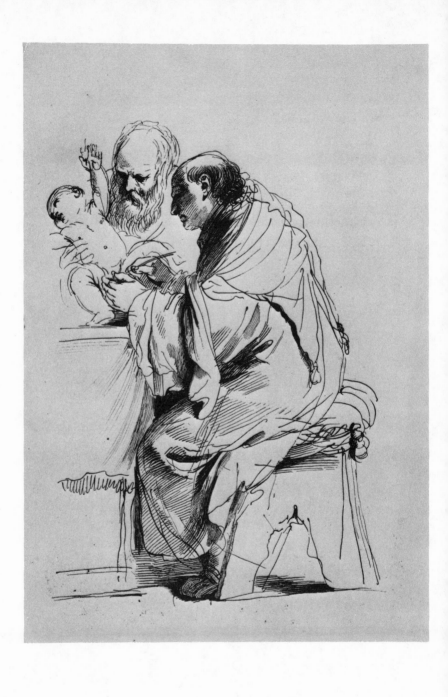

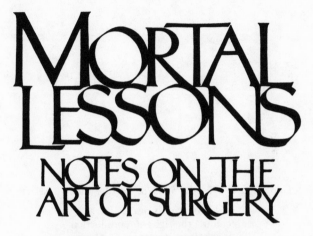

MORTAL LESSONS

NOTES ON THE ART OF SURGERY

WITH A NEW PREFACE

RICHARD SELZER

A TOUCHSTONE BOOK
Published by Simon & Schuster
New York London Toronto Sydney Tokyo Singapore

This Touchstone Edition, 1987

Published by Simon & Schuster, Inc.
Simon & Schuster Building
Rockefeller Center
1230 Avenue of the Americas
New York, New York 10020

TOUCHSTONE and colophon are registered trademarks
of Simon & Schuster, Inc.

Calligraphy by Gun Larson

Manufactured in the United States of America

7 9 10 8 6   Pbk.

Library of Congress Cataloging-in-Publication Data

Selzer, Richard.
Mortal lessons.

(A Touchstone book)
1. Surgery. I. Title.
RD39.S44   1987   617   87-4698
ISBN 0-671-64102-6 Pbk.

PREFACE

My father was a General Practitioner in Troy, New York, during the Depression. As was then the custom, his office was downstairs and we lived upstairs. At the age of ten, I took to sneaking down to his consultation room at night and there, by the light of a shame-faced candlestub, to reading the medical books on his shelves. My favorite was the *Textbook of Obstetrics and Gynecology*. It was then that I first became aware of the rich alliterative language of medicine—words such as *cerebellum* which, when said aloud, melt in the mouth and drip from the end of the tongue like chocolate. Or *carcinoma*, which sounds a lot like the aria from *Rigoletto* my mother used to sing while she washed (and I dried) the dishes. And all the rest. It should not have come as a surprise, then, that one day I would first become a doctor and then later, much later, a writer, who would try to interpret the human body and those who tend it, in the keenest language he could find.

Such a life, the life of a writing doctor, is not without its own special risk. William Butler Yeats told of Fergus, a king of Ireland, who abdicated his throne in order to learn the "dreaming wisdom"—poetry. A Druid gave Fergus a little bag of dreams—"a small slate-colored thing"—to make him forget that he ever was a king. But it did not work. Poor Fergus was suspended between the two worlds, swinging from one to the other in restless dissatisfaction. Which is about where a writing doctor is apt to find himself. The two halves of his life may be as incompatible as those of Fergus. A doctor must insulate himself against the powerful impact of mortal lessons; a writer must learn to gaze upon them with fully dilated pupils. It is not an easy thing to do both at the same time.

7

All of the pieces in this book were written in my kitchen in the middle of the night. From 1:00 A.M. to 3:00 P.M. Which is all the writing time I could spare then, my days and evenings filled with patients and surgery. I have always wondered if that shows, if the reader can tell that the book in his hand is a nocturnal creature, like a bat or an owl. Anyway, something far more likely to bite. Within these essays, stories and memoirs there are patients, nurses, doctors and others with each of whom I have, at one time or another, fallen in love. Just as any lover tries to capture and make the object of his affections his very own, so have I set my subjects down on a page and then placed them in noble or holy resonance with each other, much as the Renaissance painters did by the use of halos.

Are these characters real? the stories true? Well . . . yes and no. While each event and fact took place, while each of these people did exist, the circumstances and characters have been so filtered through my imagination as to be unrecognizable to anyone who might have been witness to them. If that seems a shortcoming to those who are bent upon getting all the facts and nothing but the facts, so be it. But facts, to one who is trying to make art, are less important than the truth that lies just beneath them waiting to be perceived. It is this truth for which the ardent writer forages among the facts, letting language lead him by the hand. To this end, I have observed the human body not only clinically, but metaphorically as well. So that the skin, and not the brain, becomes the organ of recollection, remembering the touch of a lover. A renal calculus is transformed into a philosopher's stone that lies hidden in the deepest recess of the body. A perforated peptic ulcer becomes the hole through which leaks all the rage and grief that a human being can harbor. Besides, where is it graven in stone that a writer must be unrelievedly honest? Art, by definition, is a state of sublime dishonesty. In the writing of this book I learned something about medicine and writing: they are both subcelestial arts. The angels disdain to perform either one of them.

The first section of *Mortal Lessons* is as close as I can come to realizing the art of medicine in words. In order to do this, I have used the genre of the essay, but the essay enlivened and made intimate by such fictional techniques as character, plot and dialogue. Among the news I learned in writing them is that a woman's last love affair is likely to be with her doctor; a man's last love affair is most often with his nurse. The genders, of course, being reversible. Again and again I have made use of the poetic potential of scientific description in order to illuminate an anatomical landscape.

The second section of the book constitutes an obsessive attempt to wring from language the last drop of its descriptive power, to see the body as if I had been in on its creation, or at the least, in the way Adam must have done his first lo-and-beholding in the Garden of Eden. The piece on abortion was written not to persuade the reader toward one or the other cause, but only to render the event itself in literary terms. In "The Corpse," I meant not to shock but only to step trembling into the tomb of the newly dead while holding up the lamp of language. Still, I would warn off the squeamish or those who cannot see that the truth is at least as accessible in ugliness as it is in beauty: blood spreading on a pillow, or an amputated leg that keeps still the identity of the body from which it was severed, the way a broken-off handle recalls the whole of an amphora. It could have been part of nothing else.

The last section, "Down from Troy," is a memoir of growing up in that Hudson River town that has never let go of my heart. A writer turns his back upon his native land at his own risk.

What occurs to me as I read again these essays and stories written so long ago is that surgery and writing are more alike than they are different. In surgery, it is the body that is being opened up and put back together. In writing, it is the whole world that is taken in for repairs, then put back in working order, piece by piece.

—RICHARD SELZER

CONTENTS

I

THE ART
OF SURGERY

THE EXACT
LOCATION OF THE SOUL

Someone asked me why a surgeon would write. Why, when the shelves are already too full? They sag under the deadweight of books. To add a single adverb is to risk exceeding the strength of the boards. A surgeon should abstain. A surgeon, whose fingers are more at home in the steamy gullies of the body than they are tapping the dry keys of a typewriter. A surgeon, who feels the slow slide of intestines against the back of his hand and is no more alarmed than were a family of snakes taking their comfort from such an indolent rubbing. A surgeon, who palms the human heart as though it were some captured bird.

Why should he write? Is it vanity that urges him? There is glory enough in the knife. Is it for money? One can make too much money. No. It is to search for some meaning in the ritual of surgery, which is at once murderous, painful, healing, and full of love. It is a devilish hard thing to transmit—to find, even. Perhaps if one were to cut out a heart, a lobe of the liver, a single convolution of the brain, and paste it to a page, it would speak with more eloquence than all the words of Balzac. Such a piece would need no literary style, no mass of erudition or history, but in its very shape and feel would tell all the frailty and strength, the despair and nobility of man. What? Publish a heart? A little piece of bone? Preposterous. Still I fear that is what it may require to reveal the truth that lies hidden in the body. Not all the undressings of Rabelais, Chekhov, or even William Carlos Williams have wrested it free, although God knows each one of those doctors made a heroic assault upon it.

I have come to believe that it is the flesh alone that counts. The rest is that with which we distract ourselves when we are not hungry or cold, in pain or ecstasy. In the recesses of the body I search for the philosophers' stone. I know it is there, hidden in the deepest, dampest cul-de-sac. It awaits discovery. To find it would be like the harnessing of fire. It would illuminate the world. Such a quest is not without pain. Who can gaze on so much misery and feel no hurt? Emerson has written that the poet is the only true doctor. I believe him, for the poet, lacking the impediment of speech with which the rest of us are afflicted, gazes, records, diagnoses, and prophesies.

I invited a young diabetic woman to the operating room to amputate her leg. She could not see the great shaggy black ulcer upon her foot and ankle that threatened to encroach upon the rest of her body, for she was blind as well. There upon her foot was a Mississippi Delta brimming with corruption, sending its raw tributaries down between her toes. Gone were all the little web spaces that when fresh and whole are such a delight to loving men. She could not see her wound, but she could feel it. There is no pain like that of the bloodless limb turned rotten and festering. There is neither unguent nor anodyne to kill such a pain yet leave intact the body.

For over a year I trimmed away the putrid flesh, cleansed, anointed, and dressed the foot, staving off, delaying. Three times each week, in her darkness, she sat upon my table, rocking back and forth, holding her extended leg by the thigh, gripping it as though it were a rocket that

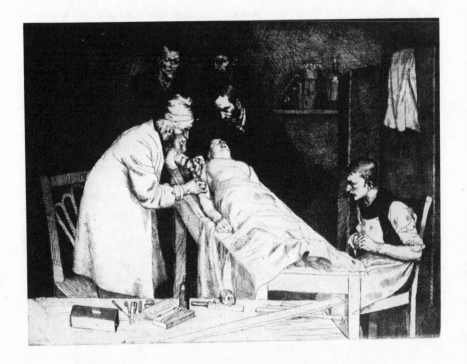

must be steadied lest it explode and scatter her toes about the room. And I would cut away a bit here, a bit there, of the swollen blue leather that was her tissue.

At last we gave up, she and I. We could no longer run ahead of the gangrene. We had not the legs for it. There must be an amputation in order that she might live—and I as well. It was to heal us both that I must take up knife and saw, and cut the leg off. And when I could feel it drop from her body to the table, see the blessed *space* appear between her and that leg, I too would be well.

Now it is the day of the operation. I stand by while the anesthetist administers the drugs, watch as the tense familiar body relaxes into narcosis. I turn then to uncover the leg. There, upon her kneecap, she has drawn, blindly, up-

17

side down for me to see, a face; just a circle with two ears, two eyes, a nose, and a smiling upturned mouth. Under it she has printed SMILE, DOCTOR. Minutes later I listen to the sound of the saw, until a little crack at the end tells me it is done.

So, I have learned that man is not ugly, but that he is Beauty itself. There is no other his equal. Are we not all dying, none faster or more slowly than any other? I have become receptive to the possibilities of love (for it is love, this thing that happens in the operating room), and each day I wait, trembling in the busy air. Perhaps today it will come. Perhaps today I will find it, take part in it, this love that blooms in the stoniest desert.

All through literature the doctor is portrayed as a figure of fun. Shaw was splenetic about him; Molière delighted in pricking his pompous medicine men, and well they deserved it. The doctor is ripe for caricature. But I believe that the truly great writing about doctors has not yet been done. I think it must be done *by* a doctor, one who is through with the love affair with his technique, who recognizes that he has played Narcissus, raining kisses on a mirror, and who now, out of the impacted masses of his guilt, has expanded into self-doubt, and finally into the high state of wonderment. Perhaps he will be a nonbeliever who, after a lifetime of grand gestures and mighty deeds, comes upon the knowledge that he has done no more than meddle in the lives of his fellows, and that he has done at least as much harm as good. Yet he may continue to pretend, at least, that there is nothing to fear, that death will not come, so long as people depend on his authority. Later, after his patients have left, he may closet himself in his darkened office, sweating and afraid.

There is a story by Unamuno in which a priest, living in a small Spanish village, is adored by all the people for his piety, kindness, and the majesty with which he celebrates the Mass each Sunday. To them he is already a saint. It is a foregone conclusion, and they speak of him as Saint Immanuel. He helps them with their plowing and planting, tends them when they are sick, confesses them, comforts them in death, and every Sunday, in his rich, thrilling voice, transports them to paradise with his chanting. The fact is that Don Immanuel is not so much a saint as a martyr. Long ago his own faith left him. He is an atheist, a good man doomed to suffer the life of a hypocrite, pretending to a faith he does not have. As he raises the chalice of wine, his hands tremble, and a cold sweat pours from him. He cannot stop for he knows that the people need this of him, that their need is greater than his sacrifice. Still . . . still . . . could it be that Don Immanuel's whole life is a kind of prayer, a paean to God?

A writing doctor would treat men and women with equal reverence, for what is the "liberation" of either sex to him who knows the diagrams, the inner geographies of each? I love the solid heft of men as much as I adore the heated capaciousness of women—women in whose penetralia is found the repository of existence. I would have them glory in that. Women are physics and chemistry. They are matter. It is their bodies that tell of the frailty of men. Men have not their cellular, enzymatic wisdom. Man is albuminoid, proteinaceous, laked pearl; woman is yolky, ovoid, rich. Both are exuberant bloody growths. I would use the defects and deformities of each for my sacred purpose of writing, for I know that it is the marred and scarred and faulty that are subject to grace. I would seek the soul in the facts of animal economy and profligacy. Yes, it is the exact location of the soul that I am after. The smell of it is in my nostrils. I have caught glimpses of it in the body diseased. If only I could tell it. Is there no mathematical equation that can guide me? So much pain and pus equals so much truth? It is elusive as the whippoorwill that one hears calling incessantly from out the night window, but which, nesting as it does low in the brush, no one sees. No one but the poet, for he sees what no one else can. He was born with the eye for it.

Once I thought I had it: Ten o'clock one night, the end room off a long corridor in a college infirmary, my last patient of the day, degree of exhaustion suitable for the appearance of a vision, some manifestation. The patient is a young man recently returned from Guatemala, from the excavation of Mayan ruins. His left upper arm wears a gauze dressing which, when removed, reveals a clean punched-out hole the size of a dime. The tissues about the opening are swollen and tense. A thin brownish fluid lips the edge, and now and then a lazy drop of the overflow spills down the arm. An abscess, inadequately drained. I will enlarge the opening to allow better egress of the pus. Nurse, will you get me a scalpel and some . . . ?

What happens next is enough to lay Francis Drake avomit in his cabin. No explorer ever stared in wilder surmise than I into that crater from which there now emerges a narrow gray head whose sole distinguishing feature is a pair of black pincers. The head sits atop a longish flexible neck arching now this way, now that, testing the air. Alternately it folds back upon itself, then advances in new boldness. And all the while, with dreadful rhythmicity, the unspeakable pincers open and close. Abscess? Pus? Never. Here is the lair of a beast at whose malignant purpose I could but guess. A Mayan devil, I think, that would soon burst free to fly about the room, with horrid blanket-wings and iridescent scales, raking, pinching, injecting God knows what acid juice. And even now the irony does not escape me, the irony of my patient as excavator excavated.

With all the ritual deliberation of a high priest I advance a surgical clamp toward the hole. The surgeon's heart is become a bat hanging upside down from his rib cage. The rim achieved—now thrust—and the ratchets of the clamp close upon the empty air. The devil has retracted. Evil mocking laughter bangs back and forth in the brain. More stealth. Lying in wait. One must skulk. Minutes pass, perhaps an hour. . . . A faint disturbance in the lake, and once again the thing upraises, farther and farther, hovering. Acrouch, strung, the surgeon is one with his instrument; there is no longer any boundary between its metal and his flesh. They are joined in a single perfect tool of extirpation. It is just for this that he was born. Now—thrust—and clamp—and *yes*. Got him!

Transmitted to the fingers comes the wild thrashing of the creature. Pinned and wriggling, he is mine. I hear the dry brittle scream of the dragon, and a hatred seizes me, but such a detestation as would make of Iago a drooling sucktit. It is the demented hatred of the victor for the vanquished, the warden for his prisoner. It is the hatred of fear. Within the jaws of my hemostat is the whole of the evil of the world, the dark concentrate itself, and I shall kill it. For mankind. And, in so doing, will open the way into a thousand years of perfect peace. Here is Surgeon as Savior indeed.

Tight grip now . . . steady, relentless pull. How it scrabbles to keep its tentacle-hold. With an abrupt moist plop the extraction is complete. There, writhing in the teeth of the clamp, is a dirty gray body, the size and shape of an English walnut. He is hung everywhere with tiny black hooklets. Quickly . . . into the specimen jar of saline . . . the lid screwed tight. Crazily he swims round and round, wiping his slimy head against the glass, then slowly sinks to the bottom, the mass of hooks in frantic agonal wave.

"You are going to be all right," I say to my patient. "We are *all* going to be all right from now on."

The next day I take the jar to the medical school. "That's the larva of the botfly," says a pathologist. "The fly usually bites a cow and deposits its eggs beneath the

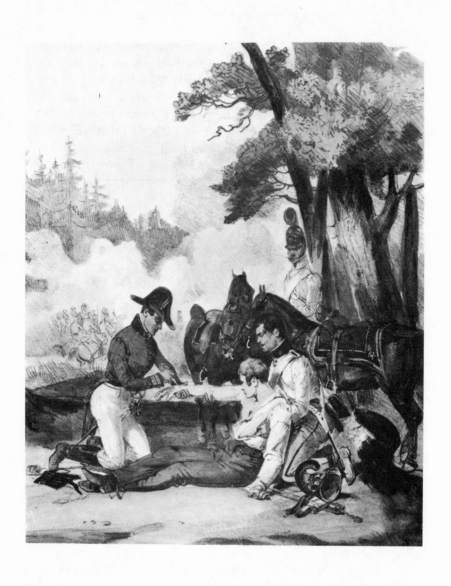

skin. There, the egg develops into the larval form which, when ready, burrows its way to the outside through the hide and falls to the ground. In time it matures into a full-grown botfly. This one happened to bite a man. It was about to come out on its own, and, of course, it would have died."

The words *imposter, sorehead, servant of Satan* spring to my lips. But now he has been joined by other scientists. They nod in agreement. I gaze from one gray eminence to another, and know the mallet-blow of glory pulverized. I tried to save the world, but it didn't work out.

No, it is not the surgeon who is God's darling. He is the victim of vanity. It is the poet who heals with his words, stanches the flow of blood, stills the rattling breath, applies poultice to the scalded flesh.

Did you ask me why a surgeon writes? I think it is because I wish to be a doctor.

THE SURGEON AS PRIEST

In the foyer of a great medical school there hangs a painting of Vesalius. Lean, ascetic, possessed, the anatomist stands before a dissecting table upon which lies the naked body of a man. The flesh of the two is silvery. A concentration of moonlight, like a strange rain of virus, washes them. The cadaver has dignity and reserve; it is distanced by its death. Vesalius reaches for his dissecting knife. As he does so, he glances over his shoulder at a crucifix on the wall. His face wears an expression of guilt and melancholy and fear. He knows that there is something wrong, forbidden in what he is about to do, but he cannot help himself, for he is a fanatic. He is driven by a dark desire. To see, to feel, to discover is all. His is a passion, not a romance.

I understand you, Vesalius. Even now, after so many voyages within, so much exploration, I feel the same sense that one must not gaze into the body, the same irrational fear that it is an evil deed for which punishment awaits. Consider. The sight of our internal organs is denied us. To how many men is it given to look upon their own spleens, their hearts, and live? The hidden geography of the body is a Medusa's head one glimpse of which would render blind the presumptuous eye. Still, rigid rules are broken by the smallest inadvertencies: I pause in the midst of an operation

24

being performed under spinal anesthesia to observe the face of my patient, to speak a word or two of reassurance. I peer above the screen separating his head from his abdomen, in which I am most deeply employed. He is not asleep, but rather stares straight upward, his attention riveted, a look of terrible discovery, of wonder upon his face. Watch him. This man is violating a taboo. I follow his gaze upward, and see in the great operating lamp suspended above his belly the reflection of his viscera. There is the liver, dark and turgid above, there the loops of his bowel winding slow, there his blood runs extravagantly. It is that which he sees and studies with so much horror and fascination. Something primordial in him has been aroused—a fright, a longing. I feel it, too, and quickly bend above his open body to shield it from his view. How dare he look within the Ark! Cover his eyes! But it is too late; he has already *seen;* that which no man should; he has trespassed. And I am no longer a surgeon, but a hierophant who must do magic to ward off the punishment of the angry gods.

I feel some hesitation to invite you to come with me into the body. It seems a reckless, defiant act. Yet there is more than dread reflected from these rosy coasts, these restless estuaries of pearl. And it is time to share it, the way the catbird shares the song which must be a joy to him and is a living truth to those who hear it. So shall I make of my fingers, words; of my scalpel, a sentence; of the body of my patient, a story.

One enters the body in surgery, as in love, as though one were an exile returning at last to his hearth, daring uncharted darkness in order to reach home. Turn sideways, if you will, and slip with me into the cleft I have made. Do not fear the yellow meadows of fat, the red that sweats and trickles where you step. Here, give me your hand. Lower between the beefy cliffs. Now rest a bit upon the peritoneum. All at once, gleaming, the membrane parts . . . and you are *in.*

It is the stillest place that ever was. As though suddenly you are struck deaf. Why, when the blood sluices fierce as Niagara, when the brain teems with electricity, and the numberless cells exchange their goods in ceaseless commerce—why is it so quiet? Has some priest in charge of these rites uttered the command "Silence"? This is no silence of the vacant stratosphere, but the awful quiet of ruins, of rainbows, full of expectation and holy dread. Soon you shall know surgery as a Mass served with Body and Blood, wherein disease is assailed as though it were sin.

Touch the great artery. Feel it bound like a deer in the might of its lightness, and know the thunderless boil of the blood. Lean for a bit against this bone. It is the only memento you will leave to the earth. Its tacitness is everlasting. In the hush of the tissue wait with me for the shaft of pronouncement. Press your ear against this body, the way you did as a child holding a seashell and heard faintly the half-remembered, longed-for sea. Now strain to listen *past* the silence. In the canals, cilia paddle quiet as an Iroquois canoe. Somewhere nearby a white whipslide of tendon bows across a joint. Fire burns here but does not crackle. Again, listen. Now there *is* sound—small splashings, tunneled currents of air, slow gaseous bubbles ascend through dark, unlit lakes. Across the diaphragm and into the chest . . . here at last it is all noise; the whisper of the lungs, the *lubdup, lubdup* of the garrulous heart.

But it is good you do not hear the machinery of your marrow lest it madden like the buzzing of a thousand coppery bees. It is frightening to lie with your ear in the pillow, and hear the beating of your heart. Not that it beats . . . but that it might stop, even as you listen. For anything that moves must come to rest; no rhythm is endless but must one day lurch . . . then halt. Not that it is a disservice to a man to be made mindful of his death, but— at three o'clock in the morning it is less than philosophy. It is Fantasy, replete with dreadful images forming in the smoke of alabaster crematoria. It is then that one thinks of the bristlecone pines, and envies them for having lasted. It is their slowness, I think. Slow down, heart, and drub on.

What is to one man a coincidence is to another a miracle. It was one or the other of these that I saw last spring. While the rest of nature was in flux, Joe Riker remained obstinate through the change of the seasons. "No operation," said Joe. "I don't want no operation."

Joe Riker is a short-order cook in a diner where I sometimes drink coffee. Each week for six months he had paid a visit to my office, carrying his affliction like a pet mouse under his hat. Every Thursday at four o'clock he would sit on my examining table, lift the fedora from his head, and bend forward to show me the hole. Joe Riker's hole was as big as his mouth. You could have dropped a plum in it. Gouged from the tonsured top of his head was a mucky puddle whose meaty heaped edge rose above the normal scalp about it. There was no mistaking the announcement from this rampart.

The cancer had chewed through Joe's scalp, munched his skull, then opened the membranes underneath—the dura mater, the pia mater, the arachnoid—until it had laid bare this short-order cook's brain, pink and gray, and pulsating so that with each beat a little pool of cerebral fluid quivered. Now and then a drop would manage the rim to run across his balding head, and Joe would reach one burry hand up to wipe it away, with the heel of his thumb, the way such a man would wipe away a tear.

I would gaze then upon Joe Riker and marvel. How dignified he was, as though that tumor, gnawing him, denuding his very brain, had given him a grace that a lifetime of good health had not bestowed.

"Joe," I say, "let's get rid of it. Cut out the bad part, put in a metal plate, and you're cured." And I wait.

"No operation," says Joe. I try again.

"What do you mean, 'no operation'? You're going to get meningitis. Any day now. And die. That thing is going to get to your brain."

I think of it devouring the man's dreams and memories. I wonder what they are. The surgeon knows all the parts of the brain, but he does not know his patient's dreams and memories. And for a moment I am tempted . . . to take the man's head in my hands, hold it to my ear, and listen. But his dreams are none of my business. It is his flesh that matters.

"No operation," says Joe.

"You give me a headache," I say. And we smile, not because the joke is funny anymore, but because we've got something between us, like a secret.

"Same time next week?" Joe asks. I wash out the wound with peroxide, and apply a dressing. He lowers the fedora over it.

"Yes," I say, "same time." And the next week he comes again.

There came the week when Joe Riker did not show up; nor did he the week after that, nor for a whole month. I drive over to his diner. He is behind the counter, shuffling back and forth between the grill and the sink. He is wearing the fedora. He sets a cup of coffee in front of me.

"I want to see your hole," I say.

"Which one?" he asks, and winks.

"Never mind that," I say. "I want to see it." I am all business.

"Not here," says Joe. He looks around, checking the counter, as though I have made an indecent suggestion.

"My office at four o'clock," I say.

"Yeah," says Joe, and turns away.

He is late. Everyone else has gone for the day. Joe is beginning to make me angry. At last he arrives.

"Take off your hat," I say, and he knows by my voice that I am not happy. He does, though, raise it straight up

with both hands the way he always does, and I see . . .
that the wound has healed. Where once there had been a
bitten-out excavation, moist and shaggy, there is now a
fragile bridge of shiny new skin.

"What happened?" I manage.

"You mean that?" He points to the top of his head. "Oh
well," he says, "the wife's sister, she went to France, and
brought me a bottle of water from Lourdes. I've been
washing it out with that for a month."

"Holy water?" I say.

"Yeah," says Joe. "Holy water."

I see Joe now and then at the diner. He looks like anything but a fleshly garden of miracles. Rather, he has taken
on a terrible ordinariness—Eden after the Fall, and minus
its most beautiful creatures. There is a certain slovenliness,
a dishevelment of the tissues. Did the disease ennoble him,
and now that it is gone, is he somehow diminished? Perhaps
I am wrong. Perhaps the only change is just the sly wink
with which he greets me, as though to signal that we have
shared something furtive. Could such a man, I think as I sip
my coffee, could such a man have felt the brush of wings?
How often it seems that the glory leaves as soon as the
wound is healed. But then it is only saints who bloom in
martyrdom, becoming less and less the flesh that pains,
more and more ghost-colored weightlessness.

It was many years between my first sight of the living
human brain and Joe Riker's windowing. I had thought
then, long ago: Could this one-pound loaf of sourdough be
the pelting brain? *This*, along whose busy circuitry run
Reason and Madness in perpetual race—a race that most
often ends in a tie? But the look deceives. What seems a
fattish snail drowzing in its shell, in fact lives in quickness,
where all is dart and stir and rapids of electricity.

Once again to the operating room . . .

How to cut a paste that is less solid than a cheese—Brie,

perhaps? And not waste any of it? For that would be a decade of remembrances and wishes lost there, wiped from the knife. Mostly it is done with cautery, burning the margins of the piece to be removed, coagulating with the fine electric current these blood vessels that course everywhere. First a spot is burned, then another alongside the first, and the cut is made between. One does not stitch—one cannot sew custard. Blood is blotted with little squares of absorbent gauze. These are called patties. Through each of these a long black thread has been sewn, lest a blood-soaked patty slip into some remote fissure, or flatten against a gyrus like a starfish against a coral reef, and go unnoticed come time to close the incision. A patty abandoned brainside does not benefit the health, or improve the climate of the intelligence. Like the bodies of slain warriors, they must be retrieved from the field, and carried home, so they do not bloat and mortify, poisoning forever the plain upon which the battle was fought. One pulls them out by their black thread and counts them.

Listen to the neurosurgeon: "Patty, buzz, suck, cut," he says. Then "Suck, cut, patty, buzz." It is as simple as a nursery rhyme.

The surgeon knows the landscape of the brain, yet does not know how a thought is made. Man has grown envious of this mystery. He would master and subdue it electronically. He would construct a computer to rival or surpass the brain. He would harness Europa's bull to a plow. There are men who implant electrodes into the brain, that part where anger is kept—the rage center, they call it. They press a button, and a furious bull halts in mid-charge, and lopes amiably to nuzzle his matador. Anger has turned to sweet compliance. Others sever whole tracts of brain cells with their knives, to mollify the insane. Here is surgery grown violent as rape. These men cannot know the brain. They have not the heart for it.

I last saw the brain in the emergency room. I wiped it

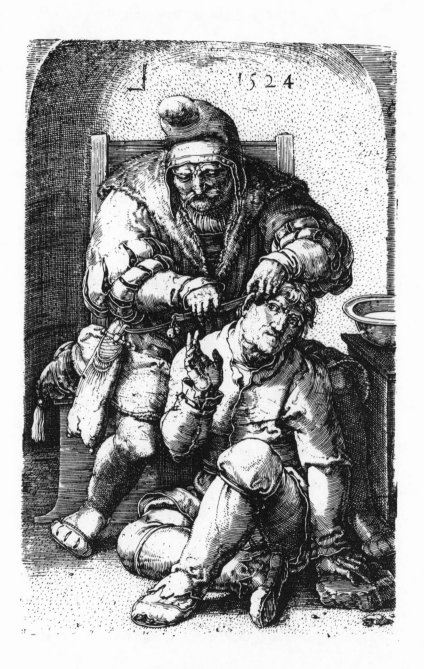

from the shoulder of a young girl to make her smashed body more presentable to her father. Now I stand with him by the stretcher. We are arm in arm, like brothers. All at once there is that terrible silence of discovery. I glance at him, follow his gaze and see that there is more brain upon her shoulder, newly slipped from the cracked skull. He bends forward a bit. He must make certain. It *is* her brain! I watch the knowledge expand upon his face, so like hers. I, too, stare at the fragment flung wetly, now drying beneath the bright lights of the emergency room, its cargo of thoughts evaporating from it, mingling for this little time with his, with mine, before dispersing in the air.

On the east coast of the Argolid, in the northern part of the Peloponnesus, lies Epidaurus. O bury my heart there, in that place I have never seen, but that I love as a farmer loves his home soil. In a valley nearby, in the fourth century B.C., there was built the temple of Asclepius, the god of medicine. To a great open colonnaded room, the abaton, came the sick from all over Greece. Here they lay down on pallets. As night fell, the priests, bearing fire for the lamps, walked among them, commanding them to sleep. They were told to dream of the god, and that he would come to them in their sleep in the form of a serpent, and that he would heal them. In the morning they arose cured. . . .

Walk the length of the abaton; the sick are in their places, each upon his pallet. Here is one that cannot sleep. See how his breath rises and falls against some burden that presses upon it. At last, he dozes, only to awaken minutes later, unrefreshed. It is toward dawn. The night lamps flicker low, casting snaky patterns across the colonnade. Already the chattering swallows swoop in and out among the pillars. All at once the fitful eyes of the man cease their roving, for he sees between the candle-lamp and the wall the shadow of an upraised serpent, a great yellow snake with topaz eyes. It slides closer. It is arched and godlike. It bends above him, swaying, the tongue and the lamplight flickering as one. Exultant, he raises himself upon one arm, and with the other, reaches out for the touch that heals.

On the bulletin board in the front hall of the hospital where I work, there appeared an announcement. "Yeshi Dhonden," it read, "will make rounds at six o'clock on the morning of June 10." The particulars were then given, followed by a notation: "Yeshi Dhonden is Personal Physician to the Dalai Lama." I am not so leathery a skeptic that I would knowingly ignore an emissary from the gods. Not only might such sangfroid be inimical to one's earthly well-being, it could take care of eternity as well. Thus, on the morning of June 10, I join the clutch of whitecoats waiting in the small conference room adjacent to the ward selected for the rounds. The air in the room is heavy with ill-concealed dubiety and suspicion of bamboozlement. At precisely six o'clock, he materializes, a short, golden, barrelly man dressed in a sleeveless robe of saffron and maroon. His scalp is shaven, and the only visible hair is a scanty black line above each hooded eye.

He bows in greeting while his young interpreter makes the introduction. Yeshi Dhonden, we are told, will examine a patient selected by a member of the staff. The diagnosis is as unknown to Yeshi Dhonden as it is to us. The examination of the patient will take place in our presence, after which we will reconvene in the conference room where Yeshi Dhonden will discuss the case. We are further informed that for the past two hours Yeshi Dhonden has purified himself by bathing, fasting, and prayer. I, having breakfasted well, performed only the most desultory of ablutions, and given no thought at all to my soul, glance furtively at my fellows. Suddenly, we seem a soiled, uncouth lot.

The patient had been awakened early and told that she was to be examined by a foreign doctor, and had been asked to produce a fresh specimen of urine, so when we enter her room, the woman shows no surprise. She has long ago taken on that mixture of compliance and resignation that is the facies of chronic illness. This was to be but another in an endless series of tests and examinations. Yeshi Dhonden steps to the bedside while the rest stand apart, watching. For a long time he gazes at the woman, favoring no part of her body with his eyes, but seeming to fix his glance at a place just above her supine form. I, too, study her. No physical sign nor obvious symptom gives a clue to the nature of her disease.

At last he takes her hand, raising it in both of his own. Now he bends over the bed in a kind of crouching stance, his head drawn down into the collar of his robe. His eyes are closed as he feels for her pulse. In a moment he has found the spot, and for the next half hour he remains thus, suspended above the patient like some exotic golden bird with folded wings, holding the pulse of the woman beneath his fingers, cradling her hand in his. All the power of the man seems to have been drawn down into this one purpose. It is palpation of the pulse raised to the state of ritual. From the foot of the bed, where I stand, it is as though he and the patient have entered a special place of isolation, of apartness, about which a vacancy hovers, and across which no violation is possible. After a moment the woman rests back upon her pillow. From time to time, she raises her head to look at the strange figure above her, then sinks back once more. I cannot see their hands joined in a correspondence that is exclusive, intimate, his fingertips receiving the voice of her sick body through the rhythm and throb she offers at her wrist. All at once I am envious—not of him, not of Yeshi Dhonden for his gift of beauty and holiness, but of her. I want to be held like that, touched so, *received*. And I know that I, who have palpated a hundred thousand pulses, have not felt a single one.

At last Yeshi Dhonden straightens, gently places the

34

woman's hand upon the bed, and steps back. The interpreter produces a small wooden bowl and two sticks. Yeshi
Dhonden pours a portion of the urine specimen into the
bowl, and proceeds to whip the liquid with the two sticks.
This he does for several minutes until a foam is raised.
Then, bowing above the bowl, he inhales the odor three
times. He sets down the bowl and turns to leave. All this
while, he has not uttered a single word. As he nears the
door, the woman raises her head and calls out to him in a
voice at once urgent and serene. "Thank you, doctor," she
says, and touches with her other hand the place he had
held on her wrist, as though to recapture something that
had visited there. Yeshi Dhonden turns back for a moment
to gaze at her, then steps into the corridor. Rounds are at
an end.

We are seated once more in the conference room. Yeshi
Dhonden speaks now for the first time, in soft Tibetan
sounds that I have never heard before. He has barely begun
when the young interpreter begins to translate, the two
voices continuing in tandem—a bilingual fugue, the one
chasing the other. It is like the chanting of monks. He
speaks of winds coursing through the body of the woman,
currents that break against barriers, eddying. These vor-
tices are in her blood, he says. The last spendings of an
imperfect heart. Between the chambers of her heart, long,
long before she was born, a wind had come and blown
open a deep gate that must never be opened. Through it
charge the full waters of her river, as the mountain stream
cascades in the springtime, battering, knocking loose the
land, and flooding her breath. Thus he speaks, and is silent.

"May we now have the diagnosis?" a professor asks.

The host of these rounds, the man who knows, answers.

"Congenital heart disease," he says. "Interventricular
septal defect, with resultant heart failure."

A gateway in the heart, I think. That must not be
opened. Through it charge the full waters that flood her

breath. So! Here then is the doctor listening to the sounds of the body to which the rest of us are deaf. He is more than doctor. He is priest.

I know . . . I know . . . the doctor to the gods is pure knowledge, pure healing. The doctor to man stumbles, must often wound; his patient must die, as must he.

Now and then it happens, as I make my own rounds, that I hear the sounds of his voice, like an ancient Buddhist prayer, its meaning long since forgotten, only the music remaining. Then a jubilation possesses me, and I feel myself touched by something divine.

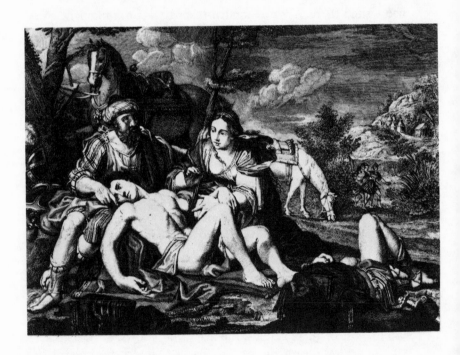

LESSONS FROM THE ART

With trust the surgeon approaches the operating table. To be sure, he is impeccably trained. He has stood here so many times before. The belly that presents itself to him this morning, draped in green linen and painted with red disinfectant, is little different from those countless others he has entered. It is familiar terrain, to be managed. He watches it rise and fall in the regular rhythm of anesthesia. Vulnerable, it returns his trust, asks but his excellence, his clever ways. With a blend of arrogance and innocence the surgeon makes his incision, expecting a particular organ to be exactly where he knows it to be. He has seen it there, in just that single place, over and again. He has aimed his blade for that very spot, found the one artery he seeks, the one vein, captured them in his hemostats, ligated them, and cut them safely; then on to the next, and the one after that, until the sick organ falls free into his waiting hand—mined.

But this morning, as the surgeon parts the edges of the wound with his retractor, he feels uncertain, for in that place where he *knows* the duct to be, there is none. Only masses of scar curtained with blood vessels of unimagined fragility. They seem to rupture even as he studies them, as though it is the abrasion of the air that breaks them. Blood is shed into the well of the wound. It puddles upon the banks of scar, concealing the way inward. The surgeon sees this, and knows that the fierce wind of inflammation has swept this place, burying the tubes and canals he seeks. It is an alien land. Now all is forestial, swampy. The surgeon suctions away the blood; even as he does so, new red trickles; his eyes are full of it; he cannot see. He advances his fingers into the belly, feeling the walls of scar, running the tips gently over each eminence, into each furrow, testing the roll of the land, probing for an opening, the smallest indentation that will accept his pressure, and invite him to follow with his instruments. There is none. It is terra incognita. Hawk-eyed, he peers, waiting for a sign, a slight change in color, that would declare the line of a tube mounding from its sunken position. There is no mark, no trail left by some earlier explorer.

At last he takes up his scissors and forceps and begins to dissect, millimetering down and in. The slightest step to either side may be the bit of excess that will set off avalanche or flood. And he is *alone*. No matter how many others crowd about the mouth of the wound, no matter their admiration and encouragement, it is *he* that rappels this crevasse, dangles in this dreadful place, and he is *afraid* —for he knows well the worth of this belly, that it is priceless and irreplaceable.

"Socked in," he says aloud. His language is astronaut terse. The others are silent. They know the danger, but they too have given him their reliance. He speaks again.

"The common bile duct is bricked up in scar . . . the pancreas swollen about it . . . soup." His voice is scarcely more than the movement of his lips. The students and interns must strain to hear, as though the sound comes from a great distance. They envy him his daring, his dexterity. They do not know that he envies them their safe footing, their distance from the pit.

The surgeon cuts. And all at once there leaps a mighty

blood. As when from the hidden mountain ledge a pebble is dislodged, a pebble behind whose small slippage the whole of the avalanche is pulled. Now the belly is a vast working lake in which it seems both patient and surgeon will drown. He speaks.

"Pump the blood in. Faster! Faster! Jesus! We are losing him."

And he stands there with his hand sunk in the body of his patient, leaning with his weight upon the packing he has placed there to occlude the torn vessel, and he watches the transfusion of new blood leaving the bottles one after the other and entering the tubing. He knows it is not enough, that the shedding outraces the donation.

At last the surgeon feels the force of the hemorrhage slacken beneath his hand, sees that the suction machine has cleared the field for him to see. He can begin once more to approach that place from which he was driven. Gently he teases the packing from the wound so as not to jar the bleeding alive. He squirts in saline to wash away the old stains. Gingerly he searches for the rent in the great vein. Then he hears.

"I do not have a heartbeat." It is the man at the head of the table who speaks. "The cardiogram is flat," he says. Then, a moment later . . . "This man is dead."

Now there is no more sorrowful man in the city, for this surgeon has discovered the surprise at the center of his work. It is death.

The events of this abdomen have conspired to change him, for no man can travel back from such darkness and be the same as he was.

As much from what happens *outside* the human body as within that place that for him has become the image of his mind, the surgeon learns.

It is Korea. 1955.

I am awakened by a hand on my chest, jostling.

"Sir Doc! Sir Doc!" It is Jang, the Korean man who assists me.

I open my eyes. Not gladly. To awaken here, in this place, in this time, is to invite despair.

"Boy come. Gate. Very scared. His brother bad sick. Pain belly. You come?"

O God, I think, let it not be appendicitis. I do not know how many more anesthesia-less operations I have left in me. Not many, I think. For I can no longer bear the gagged mouths, the trembling, frail bodies strapped to the table, round and round with wide adhesive tape from neck to ankles, with a space at the abdomen for the incision. Nor the knuckles burning white as they clutch the "courage stick" thrust into their hands at the last minute by a mamasan. Nor the eyes, slant and roving, enkindled with streaky lights. Something drags at my arms, tangles my fingers. They grow ponderous at the tips.

"Couldn't they bring him here?"

"No, Sir Doc. Too very sick."

It is midnight. I force myself to look at the boy who will guide us. He is about ten years old, small, thin, and with a festoon of snot connecting one nostril to his upper lip. It gives a harelip effect.

We are four in the ambulance: Jang, Galloway the driver, the boy, and myself. A skinny bare arm points up into the mountains where I know the road is narrow, winding. There are cliffs.

"We'll go up the stream bed," says Galloway. "It's still dry, and safer. Far as we can, then tote in."

I make none of these decisions. The ambulance responds to the commands of the boy like a huge trained beast. Who would have thought a child to have so much power in him? Soon we are in the dry gully of the stream. It is slow. Off in the distance there is a torch. It swings from side to side like the head of a parrot. A signal. We move on.

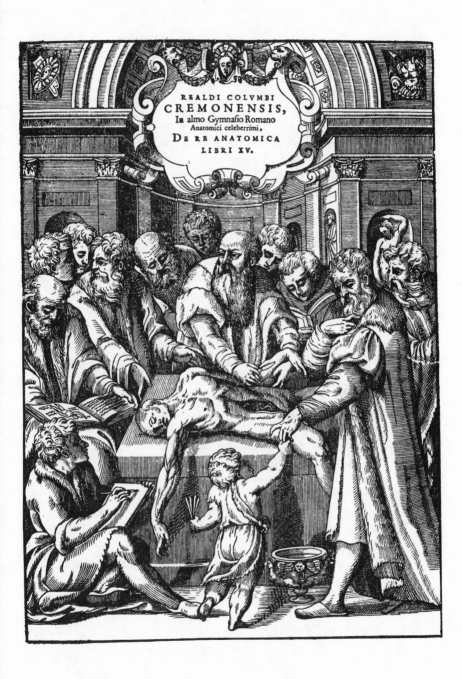

REALDI COLVMBI
CREMONENSIS,
In almo Gymnasio Romano
Anatomici celeberrimi,
DE RE ANATOMICA
LIBRI XV.

The first cool wind plays with the hair, blows the lips dry, brightens the tips of cigarettes, then skips away. In a moment it returns. Its strength is up.

"Rain start today," says Jang.

"Today?"

"Now," says Galloway. A thrum hits the windshield, spreads to the roof, and we are enveloped in rain. A flashlight floats morosely off to one side, ogling. There is shouting in Korean.

Now we are suckstepping through rice paddies, carrying the litter and tarps. We arrive at the house.

A sliding paper door opens. It is like stepping into a snail shell. On the floor mat lies a boy; he is a little smaller than the other. He wears only a loose-fitting cotton shirt out of which his head sticks like a fifth limb. His face is as tightly drawn as a fist. Flies preen there. His eyes rove in their fissures like a pendulum. I kneel. Heat rises from the skin in a palpable cloud. The ribbed bellows of the chest work above the swollen taut abdomen. Tight parts shine, I think. Knuckles and blisters and a belly full of pus. I lay my hand upon the abdomen. It helps me. I grow calm. Still, my fingers inform of the disease packaged there, swarming, lapping in untouched corners. For one moment, I long to leave it there, encased. To let it out, to cut it open, is to risk loosing it over the earth, an oceanic tide.

The abdomen is rigid, guarded. *Défense musculaire*, the French call it. You could bounce a penny on it. The slight pressure of my hand causes pain, and the child raises one translucent hand to ward me off. *Peritonitis*. Fluttering at the open lips, a single bubble expands and contracts with each breath. A soul budding there.

Outside, the sound of the rain has risen. There is anger in it. We place the boy on the litter, cover him with the tarpaulin. The door is slid open; twists of water skirl from the roof.

"Don't run," I say. "No jouncing."

The two men and the litter disappear like a melting capital H. I bow to the family of the child. Their faces are limp, flaccid; the muscles, skin, lips, eyelids—everything still. I recognize it as woe. The mother hunkers by the pallet gazing at the door. Fine colonies of sweat, like seed pearls, show upon her nose; strapped to her back, an infant twists its head away from hers in sleep. The father stands by the door. His breath is rich with kimchi; he seems to be listening. I am relieved to thrust myself into the rain.

Once again we are in the ambulance.

"The bumps," I say. "They hurt him." I need not have said that. The others knew.

There is no longer a stream bed. Where it had been, a river rushes. It has many mouths. It is maniacal. In the morning the fields below will be flooded. We drive into the torrent because . . . there is nothing else to do. We hear his little grunts, the "hic" at the end of each breath, and we enter the river. In a minute the water is at the running board, sliding back and forth on the floor. We move out to the middle. It is deeper there. In the back of the vehicle, Jang hovers over the litter, bracing it with his body. All at once, I feel the impact of the wave, like the slap of a giant tail. We are silent as the ambulance goes over on its side. We are filling with water. I push with my boots against Galloway's body, and open the door. I climb out onto the side of the ambulance.

"Pass him out. Give him here."

The moaning white figure is held up. He is naked save for the shirt. I hold him aloft. I am standing on the red cross. The others climb out. We huddle as the water screens the surface around where we stand. Then we are *in*. Rolling over and over, choking. I see the boy fly from my hands, watch him rise into the air, as in slow motion, his shirt-ends fluttering, the wind whipping the cloth. For an instant, he hangs there, his small bare arms raised, his fingers waving airily. Then he is a fish, streaking whitely, now ducking, now curving above. At last, he is a twig, turning lazily, harbored. When we reach him, he is on his back, the water rolling in and out of his mouth, his cracked head ribboning the water with blood.

All that night we walk, carrying the body in turns. The next day the father arrives. We give him the body, and I listen as Jang tells him the story of the drowning. We do not look at each other.

A man of letters lies in the intensive care unit. A professor, used to words and students. He has corrected the sentences of many. He understands punctuation. One day in his classroom he was speaking of Emily Dickinson when suddenly he grew pale, and a wonder sprang upon his face, as though he had just, for the first time, *seen* something, understood something that had eluded him all his life. It was the look of the Wound, the struck blow that makes no noise, but happens in the depths somewhere, unseen. His students could not have known that at that moment his stomach had perforated, that even as he spoke, its contents were issuing forth into his peritoneal cavity like a horde of marauding goblins. From the blackboard to the desk he reeled, fell across the top of it, and turning his face to one side, he vomited up his blood, great gouts and gobbets of it, as though having given his class the last of his spirit, he now offered them his fluid and cells.

In time, he was carried to the operating room, this man whom I had known, who had taught me poetry. I took him up, in my hands, and laid him open, and found from where he bled. I stitched it up, and bandaged him, and said later, "Now you are whole."

But it was not so, for he had begun to die. And I could not keep him from it, not with all my earnestness, so sure was his course. From surgery he was taken to the intensive care unit. His family, his students were stopped at the electronic door. They could not pass, for he had entered a new state of being, a strange antechamber where they may not go.

For three weeks he has dwelt in that House of Intensive Care, punctured by needles, wearing tubes of many calibers in all of his orifices, irrigated, dialyzed, insufflated, pumped, and drained . . . and feeling every prick and pressure the way a lover feels desire spring acutely to his skin.

In the room a woman moves. She is dressed in white. Lovingly she measures his hourly flow of urine. With hands familiar, she delivers oxygen to his nostrils and counts his pulse as though she were telling beads. Each bit of his decline she records with her heart full of grief, shaking her head. At last, she turns from her machinery to the simple touch of the flesh. Sighing, she strips back the sheet, and bathes his limbs.

The man of letters did not know this woman before. Preoccupied with dying, he is scarcely aware of her presence now. But this nurse is his wife in his new life of dying. They are close, these two, intimate, depending one upon the other, loving. It is a marriage, for although they own no shared past, they possess this awful, intense present, this matrimonial now, that binds them as strongly as any promise.

A man does not know whose hands will stroke from him the last bubbles of his life. That alone should make him kinder to strangers.

I stand by the bed where a young woman lies, her face postoperative, her mouth twisted in palsy, clownish. A tiny twig of the facial nerve, the one to the muscles of her mouth, has been severed. She will be thus from now on. The surgeon had followed with religious fervor the curve of her flesh; I promise you that. Nevertheless, to remove the tumor in her cheek, I had cut the little nerve.

Her young husband is in the room. He stands on the

opposite side of the bed, and together they seem to dwell in the evening lamplight, isolated from me, private. Who are they, I ask myself, he and this wry-mouth I have made, who gaze at and touch each other so generously, greedily? The young woman speaks.

"Will my mouth always be like this?" she asks.

"Yes," I say, "it will. It is because the nerve was cut."

She nods, and is silent. But the young man smiles.

"I like it," he says. "It is kind of cute."

All at once I *know* who he is. I understand, and I lower my gaze. One is not bold in an encounter with a god. Unmindful, he bends to kiss her crooked mouth, and I so close I can see how he twists his own lips to accommodate to hers, to show her that their kiss still works. I remember that the gods appeared in ancient Greece as mortals, and I hold my breath and let the wonder in.

Far away from the operating room, the surgeon is taught that some deaths are undeniable, that this does not deny their meaning. To *perceive* tragedy is to wring from it beauty and truth. It is a thing beyond mere competence and technique, or the handsomeness to precisely cut and stitch. Further, he learns that love can bloom in the stoniest desert, an intensive care unit, perhaps.

These are things of longest memory, and like memory, they cut. When the patient becomes the surgeon, he goes straight for the soul.

I do not know when it was that I understood that it is precisely this hell in which we wage our lives that offers us the energy, the possibility to care for each other. A surgeon does not slip from his mother's womb with compassion smeared upon him like the drippings of his birth. It is much later that it comes. No easy shaft of grace this, but the cumulative murmuring of the numberless wounds he has dressed, the incisions he has made, all the sores and ulcers and cavities he has touched in order to heal. In the begin-

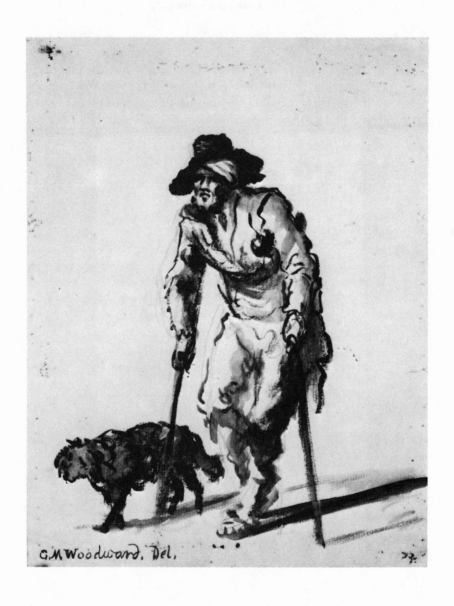

G.M.Woodward. Del.

ning it is barely audible, a whisper, as from many mouths. Slowly it gathers, rises from the streaming flesh until, at last, it is a pure *calling*—an exclusive sound, like the cry of certain solitary birds—telling that out of the resonance between the sick man and the one who tends him there may spring that profound courtesy that the religious call Love.

II

THE
BODY

BONE

Bones. Two hundred and eight of them. A whole glory turned and tooled. Lo the timbered femur all hung and strapped with beef, whose globate head nuzzles the concave underpart of the pelvis; the little carpals of the wrist faceted as jewels and as jewels named—capitate, lunate, hamate, pisiform; the phalanges, tiny kickshaws of the body, toys fantastic, worn upon the hands and feet like fans of unimagined cleverness; the porcelain pile of the vertebrae atop which rides the domed palanquin of the very brain; the vast, the slumbrous pelvis, called to wakefulness by the sweet intrusion of sex or the stirring of an impatient fetus. Out of this pelvis, endlessly rocking, drops man. I agree with those African tribes who decorate themselves with bones. It is more to my taste than diamonds, which are a cold and soulless shine. Whilst bone, ah bone, is the pit of a man after the cumbering flesh has been eaten away.

Bone is power. It is bone to which the soft parts cling, from which they are, helpless, strung and held aloft to the sun, lest man be but another slithering earth-noser. What is this tissue that has double the strength of oak? One cubic inch of which will stand a crushing force of two tons? This substance that refuses to dissolve in our body fluids, but remains intact and solid through all vicissitudes of temperature and pollution? We may be grateful for this insolubility, for it is what stands us tall. How is it that in these rigid, massive pieces is the very factory of the blood, wherein each day, one million million red blood cells are made and discharged into the circulation to course their three-score-and-one days, then die.

Stony and still though it seems, bone quickens; it flows. It is never the same at any two moments. The traverse of calcium from the blood to the bone and back again is a continuous thing, which ceaseless exchange of mineral is governed by hormonal potentates from glands afar. Fluid, too, is pressed into, then extracted from, the bone in a never-ending current, yet slow as Everglade.

In bone, as in other life, there are the givers and the takers. Twin races of cells, one the Blasts, whose function is oppositely named, for they march resolutely, all the while laying down bone, spinning out the hard stuff, each one an Atlas, born to most grittily uphold the world as he sees it. Moving steadily is the army of Clasts. These are the borers who tunnel through a bed of bone like moles through a lawn. No granitic femur is impervious to their chewings. It is not to destroy that they burrow, but to cleanse. No killers they, but peppy sweeps, clearing away old cells, all the detritus of age, the debris of ill-usage. Even as they drill their winding canaliculi, scoop out their cavitations, the rival Blasts rush in to line the spaces with new bone. Thus Blast and Clast engaged in a race between growth and decay, yet all to the single purpose of renewal. Still it must be told that it is the Clast, the devourer, that is triumphant in old age, for his energies persist, while the Blast grows weary, his deposition slow. Thus does old bone grow porous, light and brittle. Thus does it easily break, and but slowly knit.

Cartilage earns the title Mother-of-Bone. Strategically placed in the bones of the young are belts of cartilage which are the growth centers of the bone. During the first twenty years of life, this cartilage is replaced by bone at its margins even as the center remains a fiery pit of new cartilage. It must not be too hungrily replaced, before full growth is attained, or we are too short. At maturity all of the cartilage in these centers has been transformed, save for that which remains to pad the joints or, charmingly, to ornament and hold aloft the ears lest they flop like a spaniel's. In these disks of cartilage is all our stature.

Break a bone, and almost at once the blood clot between the two fragments begins to carnify. Fibrous tissue and blood vessels invade it, turn it meaty. Now, with cast or screw or metal plate, immobilize the bone so that further disruption will not take place, and the jellied mass is entered by bone-forming cells, the Blasts. Calcium salts are accepted here, and in time there is a bridge of new bone between the fragments. It is the trauma itself, the fact of fracture, that triggers the restoration. It is a cellular call to arms, a furious mobilization, an act of drive and instinct. It is the wisdom of Bone.

Remove a rib, if you must, in order to enter the chest for surgery, but leave intact the periosteum, that sheath of the bone. Strip it back, and bite away only the naked rib, and that rib will grow again, fed by the lining of the sheath, until an x-ray taken months later will reveal the marvel of the tissues. The thoracic arch has been shored up.

Bone can be grafted from one place to another to span the gap between two unhealed fragments or to fuse an unstable joint. This bone acts as a framework upon which the new bone is woven until all the pieces are joined in a single unbending whole.

No inert span this bone, but a fact of physical life each of whose parts holds a measure of electricity. Walk, and you change the electrical potential of your bones. Here it springs from positive to negative; there, from negative to positive. The strands of bone line up to follow the direction of force at any given time, seizing the position of greatest mechanical advantage, responding to each stress and shear and impact. So does it bend and relent; so does it not break; so are forgiven all the bangs and crashings of locomotion.

Like the flesh, bone is subject to defect and disease. Should the muscles attached to a bone cease to function, as in stroke or paralysis, almost half the bone served by those muscles is quickly resorbed, and disappears. Exceed the tensile strength of a bone, and it answers with the exclamation—*fracture!* Nowhere is this event more likely than in *osteogenesis imperfecta*, wherein the process of ossification is badly done. Instead of a continuing sheet of bone, there are only scanty nests of osteoblasts. An infant so afflicted may survive the trauma of birth but with half his bones broken. Merely to diaper such a child is to risk fracturing his thighs. In the aged, many small clots form in the nutrient vessels of the bone. The replenishing blood is here and there blocked, and the bone grows withered and fragile; it cracks, most often at the neck of the femur, there where the weight is borne. Such a hip fracture may be the harbinger of death for the old one forced to share his bed with Confusion and Pneumonia.

Ah, but there is more to the skull than helmet to the brain, to the sternum than shield to the heart, to the ribs than staves of the thorax. The rest of the flesh is transient, strung like laundry upon a lattice. To dwell upon bone is to contemplate the fate of man. Bone is the keepsake of the earth, all that remains of a man when the rest has long since melted and seeped and crumbled away. It endures for a million years and, if then dug up from the ground, suggests still to anthropologists the humps of meat that once it wore, and to poets the much that was from the little that remains.

What man does not ponder the whereabouts of his skeleton—the place where it will lie? Say what you will, all

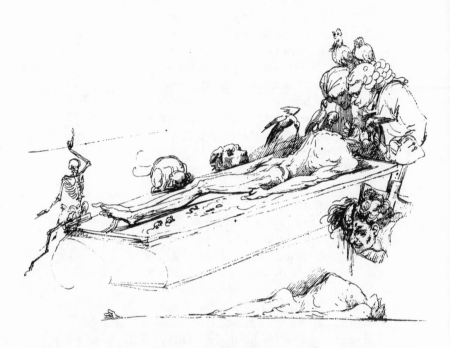

sanitary and pragmatic considerations aside, these jaunty saunterers that have held us upright, have stiffened us against the grate and grind of life, are dear to us. What stands closer to a man all his days than his bones?

A savage queen contrives from the skull of her young lover a wine bowl. Years later, as she lifts the kissed and polished calvarium to her lips, her old passion shudders anew, and licking an errant drop from one socket, she smiles in wild ownership. No thank you; not for me. Far better to tumble among the unnumbered treasures of the sea.

Of higher taste were the Ottawa Indians, friends of the explorer-priest Marquette. Upon learning the whereabouts of the body of their beloved visitor, the Ottawas journeyed there, to the eastern shore of Lake Michigan.

Journeyed eastward to the lakeside,
Where beloved pale-face rested.
Dug them up, the bones of Father,
Washed and dried them, Boxed in birch bark,
And the moon upon the waters
Lay a silver path to guide them.
Paddled chanting, in procession
Their canoes all draped in mourning,
To the chapel at the mission,
Neath the floorboards there they laid them.

Homage to Longfellow! One now understands why he wrote this way. Once you start, you can't stop.

I myself have confronted the hard fact of bone and have been changed by it. Listen.

A man named Barney died. He was my friend who sprawled face down upon rocks at the foot of a cliff. The impact had flattened and spread Barney, so that when I could scramble to where he crashed, he seemed to me wider, larger than he had been. All spaltered of limb he lay, downhill, with his head lower than his feet, his arms and legs reaching out to grapple the rocks to him, the rocks that became him so. Eagerly he had leaped, and eagerly landed.

"When I die," he had said to me that morning, "take my ashes and scatter them in this woods. Add me to this place. Do it gladly or you shall be the less for it." Barney was a hard man.

A tin can such as might be expected to hold peanuts was what the undertaker gave me, after checking the name tag. In a small clearing in the forest, where the trees leaned and interlaced above, I pried off the lid, unfolded the embossed napkin, and saw . . . not silty ash drifting and banked, but chunks of white bone the size of almonds! Here was a groove where once had ridden the trunk of a nerve; there persisted an eminence, round and smooth, to which a muscle had attached. All together they had done some act for Barney. Raised his glass, perhaps. From the can rose the faint odor of scorch. I had been ready for ash; I was filled with dread by these staring bones. From the perpetuity of ash I could have departed in peace, but from these crusts and careless crumbs, I would take away no memory of the banquet of friendship, only a nausea of the soul. Nor am I alone in my terrors. Other anatomists have touched the bones of a fellow and felt their own burial cloths winding about them. Vesalius, driven by his passion and the interdictions of society to scavenge after public hangings, poked among subgibbetal offal to retrieve yet another tibia, one fibula more. And all the while, his own heart grown ossified in his breast.

But to the task. Quickly, as though to rid myself of incriminating evidence, I walked round and round the clearing, spilling Barney's bones upon the oak leaves until there were no more. Then looked down to see them strewn as by some wizard who would read Event from the pattern in which they lay. Nearby was a small park with benches and tables and tall trash cans painted green to blend with the trees. Trembling, I went there to sit alone, for it is comforting to sit beside the dead and measure the distance between them and us.

All at once, there was a noise, an *alive* sound. Less than a thump; a scrabble perhaps. I looked behind me. There was no one, nor any creature. Only the woods where, doglike, I had dropped the bones of my friend. I sat back; again I strained toward respectful elegy. Again! A whirring. I wheeled, and . . . nothing. But now I am terrified. Who's there, I called out, and the whiteness of my voice informed the forest of my vulnerability. I started to walk away, toward the road, backing off. I must not be seized from the rear. And then I heard it again, that soft thrashing. From the rim of my vision I saw a movement. A jiggling. It was a *trash can* wobbling. Once more there was the noise, and once more the jiggling of the trash can. Now I am torn by the need to run from this demonic place and the need—yes, I must—to learn what lurks and leaps within that can that is no one-pound tin but a receptacle large enough to hold a *man*. Back and forth I flopped between resolve and panic, from No-I-shall-run-away to Stay-for-I-must. I stayed. And, stalking, crept until I had circled and sidled that horrid can three times, and heard again and again the challenge of its rattle. At last, I must act or die, and rising from a crouch, I ran full tilt toward it, kicked it with my foot high up near the top, with all my strength redoubled by fear. Over it went, rolled half a turn, and lay still. And from its gape there slouched and snarled the thinnest slice of winter I have ever seen. A raccoon. Its ribs each one visible in its flanks; its tail hairless, ignoble. Slow, contemptuous, the creature walked from the barrel. Six paces, then stopped, and turned to glare at me with loaded eyes, and lips drawn back from mauve gums, from which hung yellow teeth like tines of the gates of Hell. As I watched, the raccoon tilted back its head and loosed from its throat a sound that I shall remember all of my days. A long hiss playing out into a pneumonic rattle. It was what is left of a sigh when the rue and regret is exhausted. I felt the rank whiff upon my skin. Abruptly then, the creature walked to the edge of the woods and disappeared in the direction of the clearing where I had not gladly, not reverently thrown down the bones of my friend. I was once again alone. Barney, Barney.

Ah, you say, and smile. Spooks and banshees—childish frights. An overheated brain undoes the solid mind. Come, come, you insist. Laugh with us. And I try to join. I think fiercely of politics, of theatre, and all the stuff of daytime. But even now, years later, I start from my bed as I hear the hissing of those bones. And it does not matter what you say, or if you think that what I've told is true. It matters that I have been changed by it, that I am not the same as I was.

Does the haughty orthopedist swaggering by, tapping his boot with a pet ulna, does he pretend to a courage he does not own? Does he retreat by night to his closet quaking with fear, whilst all around his head the rumble of angry bones rolls and thunders? Or is it some fetish to which he is compelled, that he must see and touch again and again all those hard smooth strokables? For who could gaze hourly upon the bones of man and not shudder at the intimations of his mortality?

So, I have decided. No gourd, nor royal drinking cup, nor forest strew for me. Upon the wall of some quiet library ensconce my skull. Place oil and a wick in my brainpan. And there let me light with endless affection the pages of books for men to read.

Most commonly, bone is afflicted with that ubiquitous degeneration that is known as osteoarthritis, wherein the wear and tear of usage is expressed as the grinding down of the disks of cartilage that cap the ends of the bones like icing and that facilitate the movement of the joints. As the cartilage is worn thin, the joint undergoes inflammation with resultant deformity and limitation of motion. Hummocks and spurs build upon the bony surfaces, pressing against the surrounding tissues to cause pain, and thus further immobilize until the joint itself is frozen, locked, its range a pitiful semicircle or less. Live long enough, and you will win a measure of this ailment which has, more than any other, come to be synonymous with the decay of aging. That it is most apparent in the spine and hips is no more than the wages we are made to pay for the sins of our forefathers.

Of all the imprudences dared by man in his brazen reach for ascendancy, the most arrogant was his decision to stand up, to eschew his all-fours, and, piling his vertebrae one atop the other, to thrust himself erect. Admittedly, there were prizes to be won by this recklessness. An apple, heretofore waggling from a branch just out of reach, could now be plucked with ease. Ledges and rocks which had, up to then, walled him in could now be overpeered. Prey could be seen advancing; enemies too, long before their arrival. And rocks could be flung farther from the new height. Most exhilarating was the discovery of front-to-front copulation, a stunning innovation that ushered in the process of selection of a mate, now euphemistically called love. Prior to his standing up, man, like the others, copulated front-to-back, nor did it matter whose front, whose back. Now, laughing himself sick at kine and behemoth, *Homo erectus* picked and chose. This one had nice furry breasts; that one was gimpy. This one was bald; that, one-eyed. Having chosen, and wishing to keep the good parts in view, bifrontal copulation seemed but the natural sequitur. Woman, in her turn, was rewarded with orgasm, a phenomenon unknown to all other species.

It all seemed like such a good idea.

But this man who thrust himself from the earth, who wore the stars of heaven in his hair, was guilty of overweening pride. In act most audacious, he had defied nothing less than the law of gravity. He was to pay dearly for such high imposture. The vertebrae, unused to their new columnar arrangement, slipped, buckled, and wore out. Next, the arches of the feet fell. The hip joints ground to a halt. Nor was payment extorted only from the skeletal system. The pooling of blood in the lower part of the body distended the fragile blood vessels beyond their limits. Thus bloomed the fruitage of hemorrhoids; thus are we varicose. Worse still, our soft underparts have given way. Under the sag of our guts, we bulge into hernia. We turn to soft lump.

Alas, was there no pithecanthropoid Jeremiah who, horrified at the vainglory of the young, would scramble to some lofty place and cry out against this swagger? Would cry out to his fellow man, "Down, you fools. Get down, before it is too late"? So we have come to our pretty pass. Better to have maintained our low profile, content to nose among the droppings of mastodons—for it is swollen, bunched, sacculent, hung down, gibbous, hummocky, knobbed, sagging, adroop, warped, tipped, and tilted, that we are made to wage life, slouching toward our infernal copulations and our eternal reward. Such is the revenge of bone.

LIVER

What is the size of a pumpernickel, has the shape of Diana's helmet, and crouches like a thundercloud above its bellymates, turgid with nourishment? What has the industry of an insect, the regenerative powers of a starfish, yet is turned to a mass of fatty globules by a double martini (two ounces of alcohol)? It is . . . the liver, doted upon by the French, assaulted by the Irish, disdained by the Americans, and chopped up with egg, onion, and chicken fat by the Jews.

Weighing in at three to four pounds, about one fiftieth of the total body heft, the liver is the largest of the glands. It is divided into two great lobes, the right and left, and two small lobes, the caudate and the quadrate, spitefully named to vex medical students. In the strangely beautiful dynamism of embryology, the liver appears as a tree that grows out of the virgin land of the foregut in order to increase its metabolic and digestive function. Its spreading crown of tissue continues to draw nourishment from the blood vessels of the intestine. Legion are the functions of this workhorse, the most obvious of which is the manufacture and secretion of a pint of bile a day, without which golden liquor we could not digest so much as a single raisin; and therefore, contrary to the legend that the liver is an organ given to man for him to be bilious with, in its absence we should become rather more cantankerous and grouchy than we are.

I think it altogether unjust that as yet the liver has failed to catch the imagination of modern poet and painter as has the heart and more recently the brain. The heart is purest theatre, one is quick to concede, throbbing in its cage palpably as any nightingale. It quickens in response to the emotions. Let danger threaten, and the thrilling heart skips a beat or two and tightrope-walks arrhythmically before lurching back into the forceful thump of fight or flight. And all the while we feel it, hear it even—we, its stage and its audience.

One will grant the heart a modicum of history. Ancient man slew his enemy, then fell upon the corpse to cut out his heart, which he ate with gusto, for it was well understood that to devour the slain enemy's heart was to take upon oneself the strength, valor and skill of the vanquished. It was not the livers or brains or entrails of saints that were lifted from the body in sublimest autopsy, it was the heart, thus snipped and cradled into worshipful palms, then soaked in wine and herbs and set into silver reliquaries for the veneration of the faithful. It follows quite naturally that Love should choose such an organ for its bower. In the absence of Love, the canker gnaws it; when Love blooms therein, the heart dances and *tremor cordis* is upon one.

As for the brain, it is all mystery and memory and electricity. It is enough to know of its high-topping presence, a gray cloud, substantial only in the bony box of the skull and otherwise melting into a blob of ghost-colored paste that can be wiped up with a sponge. The very idea of it, teeming with a billion unrealized thoughts, countless circuits breaking and unbreaking, flashing tiny fires of idea on and off, is too much. One bows before the brain, fearing, struck dumb. Or almost dumb, saying pretty things like, "The brain is wider than the sky," or silly things like, "The brain secretes thought as the stomach gastric juice, the kidneys urine." Or this: "Rest, with nothing else, corrodes the brain," which is a damnable lie.

It is time to turn aside from our misplaced meditation on the privileged brain, the aristocratic heart. Let the proletariat arise. I give you . . . the liver! Let us celebrate that great maroon snail, whose smooth back nestles in the dome of the diaphragm, beneath the lattice of the rib cage, like some blind wise slave, crouching above its colleague viscera, secret, resourceful, instinctive. No wave of emotion sweeps it. Neither music nor mathematics gives it pause in its appointed tasks. Consider first its historical role.

Medicine, as is well known, is an offshoot of religion. The predecessor of the physician as healer was the priest as exorciser. It is a quite manageable leap for me from demons to germs as the source of disease. It is equally easy to slide from incantation to prescription. Different incantations for different diseases, I gather, and no less mysterious to the ancient patients than the often mystic formulae of one's family doctor. The mystery was and is part of it. Along with the priest as exorciser was the priest as diviner, who was able to forestall illness by his access to the wishes of the gods, a theory that has since broadened into the field of preventive medicine. The most common method of divination was the inspection of the liver of a sacrificial animal, as is documented in cultures ranging from the Babylonian through the Etruscan to the Greek and Roman. Why the liver as the "organ of revelation par excellence"? Well, here it is:

In the beginning it was the liver that was regarded as the center of vitality, the source of all mental and emotional activity, nay, the seat of the soul itself. Quite naturally, the gods spoke therein. What a gloriously hepatic age! A man could know when and how best to attack his enemy, whether his amorous dallying would bring joy unemcumbered with disease, whether the small would be great, the great laid low. All one had to do was to drag a sheep to the temple, flip a drachma to an acolyte, and stand by while the priests slit open the belly and read the markings of the liver, the position of the gallbladder, the arrangement of the ducts and lobes. It was all there, in red and yellow. This sort of thing went on for three thousand years and, one might ask, what other practice has enjoyed such longevity? Even so recent a personality as Julius Caesar learned of the bad vibes of the Ides of March from an old liver lover, although that fellow used a goat instead of a sheep, and a purist might well have been skeptical. Incidentally, the reason the horse was never used for divination is that it is difficult to lift onto altars, and also does not possess a gallbladder, a fact of anatomy that has embarrassed and impoverished veterinarians through the ages.

It was only with the separation of medicine from the apron strings of religion and the rise of anatomy as a study in itself that the liver was toppled from its central role and the heart was elevated to the chair of emotions and intellect. The brain is even more recently in the money, and still has not quite overcome the heart as the seat of the intellect, as witness the quaint reference to learning something "by heart." Soon the heart was added to the organs used for prophecy by the Greeks and Romans, who then threw in the lungs, and finally, with an overdeveloped sense of organic democracy, the intestines. Since the liver was no longer *the* divine organ in the animal, out it transited along with Ozymandias and other sic glorias, which decline so dispirited the hepatoscopists that soon they gave up the whole damned rite and went off to listen sulkily to Hippocrates rhapsodize, tastelessly I think, about the brain and heart. As if that were not bad enough, Plato placed the higher emotions, such as courage, squarely above the diaphragm, and situated the baser appetites below, especially in the liver, where they squat like furry beasts even today, as is indicated in the term "lily-livered," or "choleric," or worse, "bilious." The assassination was complete. Still, there are memories, and the sense of history is a power and glory to all but the most swinish of men.

Today all that is left of the practice of divination is the unofficial cult of phrenology, in which character is interpreted from the bumps of the skull, and the science of palmistry, which is a rather ticklish business to get into, and seems to me merely a vulgar attempt to transfer divination to a more accessible part of the body. Nevertheless, my palmist always places great emphasis on the length and curve of the hand marking known as the "line of the liver."

The closest thing to liver worship still in business is the reverent sorrow with which the French regard their beloved *foie*. It is at once recalcitrant child and stern paterfamilias. This national preoccupation is entirely misunderstood, and thus held in ill-deserved contempt by the rest of the world, which regards such hepatism as a form of mass hypochondria. In fact, it is wholly admirable after the shallow insouciance and hectic swilling of the Americans, for instance. The French understand the absolute fairness of life, that if you want to dance you have to pay the fiddler. Nothing in our country so binds the populace into a single suffering fraternity, any of whose members has but to raise his eyebrows and tap himself below the ribs to elicit a heartfelt moue of commiseration from a passing stranger. In the endless discussions of the relative merits of the various mineral waters, or whether the cure taken at Vichy or Montecatini effects a more enduring remission, class distinctions become as vague as mist. Princes of the Church, Communists at the barricade, légionnaires d'honneur, and chimney sweeps lock hearts and arms in the thrill of fellowship. Napoleon himself, wintering bitterly near Moscow in 1812, yearned not for Paris, or the Seine, or Versailles, or even for Josephine, but for Vichy and *the cure*. Obviously it is in the camaraderie of the liver and not in fragile treaties or grudging coexistence that the hope of the world lies—

for ardently though one might wish to wash the brain of one's enemy, to bomb, bug or hijack him, never would one sink to the infliction of harm upon his liver.

That these same French viciously funnel great quantities of grain into the stomachs of their geese in order to fatten the livers for pâté de foie gras, I consider simply a regrettable transference of their own hepatic anxiety onto their poultry. It is as though by bringing on such barnyard *crises de foie* they are in some way exorcised of their own. Ah, the power of insight! To gain it is to forgive and to love.

Deplorable is the constipated English view, delivered with nasal sanctimony, that the Continental liver phobia is an old wives' tale. One has but to glance at any recent map of the British Empire to know the folly of this opinion. Equally regrettable is the *que sera, sera* attitude in the United States, where the last homage to the liver was paid by the faithful users of Carter's Little Liver Pills, until the federal government invaded even that small enclave of devotion by ordering the discontinuance of the word "Liver." Now, oh, God, it's just plain Carter's Little Pills and we are the poorer.

Man's romance with alcohol had its origins in the Neolithic Age or earlier, presumably from the accidental tasting by some curious fellow of, let's say, fermented honey, or mead as it is written in *Beowulf*. The attainment of the resultant euphoria has remained a continuous striving of the human race with the exception of the perverse era of Prohibition, which presumed to tear asunder that which Nature had joined in absolute harmony. Even in the Scriptures it is implied that Noah had a lot to drink, and Lot could not say Noah. From its first appearance on the planet, alcohol has never been absent from the scene. An early hieroglyphic of the Eighteenth Egyptian Dynasty has a woman calling out for eighteen bowls of wine. "Behold," she cries, "I love drunkenness."

The human body is perfectly suited for the ingestion of alcohol, and for its rapid utilization. In that sense we are not unlike alcohol lamps. Endless is our eagerness to devour alcohol. Witness the facts that it is absorbed not only from the intestine, as are all other foods, but directly from the stomach as well. It can be taken in by the lungs as an inhalant, and even by the rectum if given as an enema. Once incorporated into the body, it is to the liver that belongs the task of oxidizing the alcohol. But even the sturdiest liver can handle only a drop or two at a time, and the remainder swirls ceaselessly about in the bloodstream, is exhaled by the lungs and thus provides the state police with a crackerjack method of detecting and measuring the presence and amount of alcohol ingested. Along the way it bathes the brain with happiness, lifting the inhibitory cortex off the primal swamp of the id and permitting to surface all sorts of delicious urges such as the one to walk into people's houses wearing your wife's hat. Happily enough, the brain is not organically altered by alcohol unless taken in near-lethal amounts. The brain cells are not destroyed by it in any kind of moderate drinking, and if the alcohol is withdrawn from the diet, the brain rapidly awakens and resumes its function at the usual, if not normal, level. One must reckon, nevertheless, with the hangover, which retributive phenomenon is devised to make the drinker feel guilty. In fact, it is not more than a nightmarish echo of the state of inebriation brought on by excessive fatigue and the toxic effects of congeners, the natural products of the fermentation process that give distinction to the taste of the various forms of alcohol. In *The Adventures of Huckleberry Finn*, we find Huck awakening to "an awful scream. . . . There was pap looking wild, and skipping around every which way, and yelling about snakes. He said they was crawling up his legs; and then he would give a jump and scream, and say one had bit him on the cheek—but I couldn't see no snakes. He started and run round and

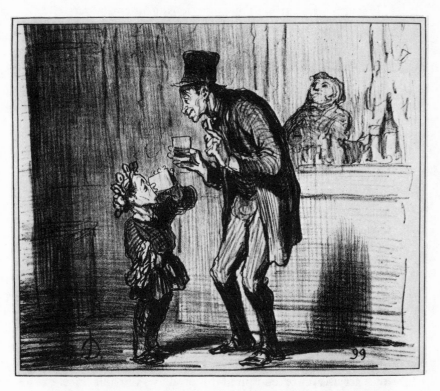

round the cabin, hollering. 'Take him off. Take him off; he's biting me on the neck!' I never see a man look so wild in the eyes. Pretty soon he was all fagged out, and fell down panting; then he rolled over and over wonderful fast, kicking things every which way, and striking and grabbing at the air with his hands, and screaming, and saying there was devils ahold of him. He wore out by and by, and laid still awhile, moaning. Then he laid stiller, and didn't make a sound."

It was a French physician, quite naturally, who first de-scribed the disease known as cirrhosis of the liver, near the turn of the nineteenth century. His name, René Théophile

Hyacinthe Laënnec. This fastidious gentleman was the very same whose aversion to applying his naked ear to the perfumed but unbathed bosoms of his patients inspired him to invent the stethoscope, which idea he plagiarized from a group of street urchins playing with rolled-up paper. The entire medical world continues to pay homage to Laënnec for his gift of space interpersonal. As if this were not enough, he permitted himself to be struck by the frequent appearance at autopsy of livers that were yellow, knobby and hard. This marvel he named cirrhosis, from the Greek word for tawny, *kirrhos*. The liver appears yellow because it is fatty, hard because it is scarred, and knobby because the regeneration of liver tissue between the scars produces little mounds or hillocks. It was suspected by Laënnec, and is known by all the rest of us today, that by far the most common cause of cirrhosis is the consumption of alcohol.

It is a matter for future anthropologists to ponder that the two favorite companions of business are Bottle and Board. More than one eminent literary agent, Wall Street broker, and vice-president have died testifying affection for them. Deep drinking and intrigue are part of all the noble professions. These, combined with the studious avoidance of exercise, have conspired to produce a whole race of voluptuaries who, by twos and threes from noon till three, sit at tables in dim restaurants, picking at their sideburns and destroying the furniture with their gigantic buttocks. These same men can be seen after five years of such indiscretion transformed into "lean and slippered pantaloons," with scanty hair that is but the gray garniture of premature senescence.

In the city of New York such is the torrent of spirituous flow as to make the clinking of ice cubes and the popping of corks a major source of noise pollution. It is as though it had been purported by the Surgeon General himself that the best means of maintaining human life from infancy to extreme old age were by the copious use of the Blood of the Grape. It might with equal credibility be put forth that tobacco smoke purifies the air from infectious malignancy by its fragrance, sweetens the breath, strengthens the brain and memory, and restores admiration to the sight.

Counting every man, woman and child in the United States, it is estimated that the average daily intake of calories is thirty-three hundred a person. In this all-inclusive group, one hundred sixty-five calories are ingested as alcohol. Pushing on, if one were to divide these Americans into I Do Drinks and I Don't Drinks, the I Do's take in five hundred calories from this same source. This alcohol is metabolized in the liver by a fiercely efficient enzyme called alcohol dehydrogenase, and transformed directly into energy, which would all be terribly nice were it not for the unjust fact that alcohol is poisonous to the liver, causing it to become loaded with fat. If enough is imbibed, and enough fat is deposited in the liver, this organ takes on the yellowish color noted by Laënnec. Still more booze, and the liver becomes heavy with fat, swelling so that it emerges from beneath the protective rib cage and bulges down into the vulnerable soft white underbelly. There it can be palpated by the examining fingers, and even seen protruding on the right side of the abdomen in some cases.

Even today, the progression from this fatty stage to the frank inflammation and scarring that are the hallmarks of cirrhosis is not well understood. Factors other than continued drinking pertain here. One of these is susceptibility. Jews, for instance, are not susceptible. One sees precious few cirrhotic Jews. It was formerly averred by somewhat chauvinistic Jewish hepatologists that Jews didn't get cirrhosis because they didn't drink much, what with their strong, dependable family ties, and their high motivation, and their absolute need to excel in order to survive. They didn't need to drink. But Jews are now among the most emancipated of drinkers and, with all the fervor of new converts, are causing such virtuosi as the Irish and the

French to glance nervously over their shoulders. Still, the Jews do not get cirrhosis. This is not to say that they are not alcoholics. It has been reported by more than one visiting professor of medicine that noticeable segments of the population of Israel get and stay drunk for quite heroic periods of time. It is also reported that their livers remain enviably healthy.

Another measure of susceptibility is, brace yourselves, the absence of hair on the chest. In males, of course. Unpelted men of the sort idealized by bathing-suit and underwear manufacturers are sitting ducks for the onset of cirrhosis. All other things being equal, women, the marrying kind, would do well to turn aside from such vast expanses of naked chest skin and to cultivate a taste for the simian. It was formerly thought that cirrhotic men lost their chest hair. Not so. They never had any to begin with.

Lastly, it is said by some that climate is a factor: the closer to the equator, the more vulnerable the liver. Thus, a quantity of alcohol that scarcely ruffles the frozen current of a Norwegian's blood would scatter madness and fever into the brain of a Hindu.

There is a difference, I hasten to add, between imbibers of alcohol and alcoholics. Both develop fatty livers, true, but no one has shown conclusively that a fatty liver is the precursor of cirrhosis. One martini increases the fat content of the liver sufficiently so that it can be seen by the use of special stains under the microscope. In other words, a single martini increases the fat in a liver by one half percent of the weight of the organ, above a normal three percent. In the alcoholic this commonly reaches a death-defying twenty-five percent. But you don't have to be an alcoholic to get cirrhosis. Some quite modest drinkers get it. Nor does it matter the purity of the spirits consumed. Beer, wine, and whiskey equally offend, and he who would take comfort from the idea that he drinks only beer, or only wine, is to be treated with pity and contempt. One correlation that does hold water is the duration of time that one has been drinking. Cirrhosis is primarily a disease of the forties or fifties. Even here we cannot generalize, however, for great numbers of younger people are afflicted, and one patient within my ken was an eighteen-year-old girl whose voluminous liver could be felt abutting on her groin just eight months after she had retired to her room with a continuous supply of Thunderbird wine.

The state of nutrition is also a factor in the development of cirrhosis. It is no secret that boozers, the serious kind, stop eating, especially protein, either because they can't afford it—what with the cost of a bottle of bourbon these days—or because the sick liver just can't handle the metabolism of protein well, and the appetite is warned off.

The nitrogenous material of protein passes directly through the diseased liver and exerts a toxic effect on the brain. If one restricts protein in the diet of cirrhotics, the brain improves. A case in point is Sir Andrew Aguecheek of *Twelfth Night,* whose fervent wish to cut a dash was aborted by stupidity, cowardice, and social gaucherie. His eccentricity, emotional lability and restricted vocabulary were almost certainly due to the organic brain syndrome of liver disease due to intolerance of nitrogen. Sir Toby Belch assesses Sir Andrew rather highly. Still, Sir Toby cannot resist the clinical judgment that "For Andrew, if he were opened, and you find so much blood in his liver as will clog the foot of a flea, I'll eat the rest of the anatomy." Such as Sir Andrew Aguecheek are thrown into mental confusion, confabulation and even coma by no more than a single ounce of beef. Thus their medical nickname, "one meatballers."

In an analysis of the inhabitants of Chicago's Skid Row, it was observed that a customary diet consisted of alcohol in any form and jelly doughnuts. Yet in the cases of thirty-nine hundred such folk whose death certificates were signed out as cirrhosis, only ten percent were actually found to have the disease at autopsy. Thus it might be stated that alcoholics exceed cirrhotics by nine to one—or that only ten percent of alcoholics get cirrhosis.

What is clearly needed is a test to find out which are the ten percent that are going to get it, so that the rest of us can enjoy ourselves. At the moment I prefer to take comfort from the example of such valiant topers as Winston Churchill, who swallowed a fifth of whiskey a day all the while leading Great Britain in her finest hour, and went on to die in his nineties, still holding his fingers up like that. It is also true that if one, moved by some transcendental vision or goaded by ill-conceived guilt, abstains from further drinking, in short order all the excess fat departs from the liver and it once again regains its pristine color and size. In this way do spree drinkers inadvertently rest their livers and avoid the cirrhosis we slow but steadies risk. Thus something can be said for periodic abstinence, a wisdom one would hesitate to translate into other vices.

Before enumerating the signs and symptoms of cirrhosis, and thus running the risk of offending sensibility, it should be unequivocally affirmed that he is no gentleman, in fact a very milksop, of no bringing up, that will not drink. He is fit for no company, for it is a credit to have a strong brain and carry one's liquor well. Saith Pliny, " 'Tis the greatest good of our tradesmen, their felicity, life and soul, their chiefest comfort, to be merry together in a tavern."

Envision, if you will, a house whose stones are living hexagonal tiles not unlike those forming the bathroom floors of first-class hotels. These are the hepatocytes, the cellular units of the liver. Under the microscope they have a singular uniformity, each as like unto its fellow as the antlers of a buck, and all fitted together with a lovely imprecision so as to form a maze of crooked hallways and oblong rooms. Coursing through this muralium of tissue are two arborizations of blood vessels, the one bringing food and toxins from the intestine, the other delivering oxygen from the heart and lungs. Winding in and among these networks is a system of canaliculi that puts to shame all the aqueductal glories of Greece and Rome. Through these sluice the rivers of bile, gathering strength and volume as the little ducts at the periphery meet others, going into ones of larger caliber, which in turn fuse, and so on until there are two large tubes emerging from the undersurface of the liver. Within this magic house are all the functions of the liver carried out. The food we eat is picked over, sorted out, and stored for future use in the cubicles of the granary. Starch is converted to glycogen, which is released in the form of energy as the need arises. Protein is broken down into its building blocks, the amino acids, later to be fashioned into more YOU, as old tissues die off and need to be replaced. Fats are stored until sent forth to provide warmth and comfort. Vitamins and antibodies are released into the bloodstream. Busy is the word for the liver. Deleterious substances ingested, inadvertently like DDT or intentionally like alcohol, are either changed into harmless components and excreted into the intestine, or stored in locked closets to be kept isolated from the rest of the body. Even old blood cells are pulverized and recycled. Such is the ole catfish liver snufflin' along at the bottom of the tank, sweepin', cleanin' up after the gouramis, his whiskery old face stirrin' up a cloud of rejectimenta, and takin' care of everything.

But there are limits. Along comes that thousandth literary lunch and—Pow! the dreaded wrecking ball of cirrhosis is unslung. The roofs and walls of the hallways, complaining under their burden of excess fat, groan and buckle. Inflammation sets in, and whole roomfuls of liver cells implode and die, and in their place comes the scarring that twists and distorts the channels, pulling them into impossible angulation. Avalanches block the flow of bile and heavy tangles of fiber impede the absorption and secretion.

This happens not just in one spot but all over, until the gigantic architecture is a mass of sores and wounds, the old ones scarring over as new ones break down.

The obstructed bile, no longer able to flow down to the gut, backs up into the bloodstream to light up the skin and eyes with the sickly lamp of jaundice. The stool turns toothpaste white in commiseration, the urine dark as wine. The belly swells with gallons of fluid that weep from the surface of the liver, no less than the tears of a loyal servant so capriciously victimized. The carnage spreads. The entire body is discommoded. The blood fails to clot, the palms of the hands turn mysteriously red, and spidery blood vessels leap and crawl on the skin of the face and neck. Male breasts enlarge, and even the proud testicles turn soft and atrophy. In a short while impotence develops, an irreversible form of impotence which may well prod the invalid into more and more drinking.

Scared? Better have a drink. You look a little pale. In any case there is no need to be all that glum. Especially if you know something that I know. Remember Prometheus? That poor devil who was chained to a rock, and had his liver pecked out each day by a vulture? Well, he was a classical example of the regeneration of tissue, for every night his liver grew back to be ready for the dreaded diurnal feast. And so will yours grow back, regenerate, reappear, regain all of its old efficiency and know-how. All it requires is quitting the booze, now and then. The evergrateful, forgiving liver will respond joyously with a multitude of mitoses and cell divisions that will replace the sick tissues with spanking new nodules and lobules of functioning cells. This rejuvenation is carried on with the speed and alacrity of a starfish growing a new ray from the stump of the old. New channels are opened up, old ones dredged out, walls are straightened and roofs shored up. Soon the big house is humming with activity, and all those terrible things I told you happen go away—all except that impo-

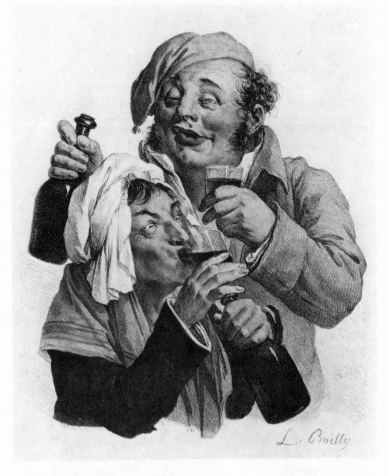

tence thing. Well, you didn't expect to get away scot-free, did you?

And here's something to tuck away and think about whenever you want to feel good. Sixty percent of all cirrhotics who stop drinking will be alive and well five years later. How unlike the lofty brain which has no power of regeneration at all. Once a brain cell dies, you are forever one shy.

Good old liver!

STONE

Delicate durability describes the human body, and nowhere is this more apparent than in the urinary tract. If the liver is all bulk and thunder, the heart fist and thrust and piston, and the brain a foamy paste of insubstantial electricity, the parts of the urinary tract—namely the kidneys, ureters, and bladder—are a tracery of tubules and ducts of such a fineness as would lay mad a master plumber, more, a Venetian glassblower. Lifted whole from the magic forest of the body and considered apart, the organs of urination resemble the head of a strangely sweet-faced creature. Here are the twin ears of the kidneys, blooming above the slender ureteral stalks. They are paired bean-shaped organs, together weighing less than one pound, that lie on either side of the spine behind the other organs. The right is somewhat lower than the left, being sat upon by the monopolizing bulk of the liver, and each is protected by the lowermost ribs. Both wear, with Napoleonic panache, the tricornered hat of the adrenal gland.

The ureters, a foot or more in length, are drawn out to the finest filaments before joining the bowl of the bladder. This virtuoso fills passively, until, aroused by its own tidal volume, it contracts in vigorous expression. From its nethermost surface, the tapered spout of the urethra extends to deliver to the out-of-doors the jet of urine that is the raison d'être of the whole mechanism.

The business of this system is the collection and excretion of the liquid wastes of the body. The production of urine is continuous. Consider the magnitude of the task. Between three and one half and six quarts of blood, one fifth of the total pumped by the heart each minute, are passed immediately to the kidneys, where the stream of blood is thinned out into two million tiny rivulets, each still possessed of some of the high pressure provided by the force of the heartbeat. The tiny arteries within the substance of the kidney come in contact with the equally tiny tubules of the urine-collecting system within microscopic knobs called glomerular tufts. Here, the higher pressure of the blood pushes the waste products across the thin vessel walls into the fragile tubules, whose low pressure puts up no resistance and which accept quite passively the materials —salt, water and impurities—that go to make up the urine. One hundred and eighty quarts a day are filtered across these membranes in order to produce one and a half quarts of urine. Thus, ninety-nine and two tenths percent of the filtered water is reabsorbed by the tubular system of the kidney and sent back into the body, and we do not die of immediate dehydration. With equal precision, most of the salts are reabsorbed, only a trifling amount finally being excreted. In addition to the filtrative and reabsorptive functions of the kidney, the cells of the tubules are capable of excreting waste themselves, adding to the stream of sewage even as they tunnel it toward the next compartment. All this to maintain what Claude Bernard, the great French physiologist, called our *internal environment*. Truly, the kidney is the organ of discrimination.

Once clear of the kidney, the urine flows down the ureters, squeezed toward the bladder by the writhing contractility of these tubes and the fanning downward of the cilia that project from the lining. In the bladder, that most gifted of muscular bottles, commodious to the amount of two quarts under extreme circumstances, the urine is collected until approximately one half pint is present, whereupon the pressure signal is given, discharged to the brain, and the order returned. All at once the great detrusor muscle grinds inward, pushing downward symmetrically toward the urethra, which strait is guarded by a circular sphincter, closed during the long filling period, but now suddenly thrown open to allow the forceful flow of urine into the urethra and to the outside. And you thought you were just passing your water!

Perhaps not without a touch of irony, the excretory function is housed in tissues adjacent to those of reproduction, even to the extent of sharing the final pathways of discharge. Although to certain fastidious creatures this might seem the cruelest of jokes, it would be difficult to imagine a more appropriate and less acrobatically inconvenient location for each, when all is said and done. Examined in another light, this systemic neighborliness serves to humble the human race.

Still, there is some risk in this proximity of the genital and urinary systems, for the base of the male urethra is guarded by the twin rocks of the prostate. This organ, a look-alike of the turkey gizzard, has for its function the production and discharge of the fluid in which the sperm are carried to their ultimate destination. One of the more regrettable of the changes of the aging process is the slow, inexorable enlargement and hardening of the prostate, causing it to project more and more deeply into the urethral canal. The urinary stream becomes dismayingly slow. There is hesitancy in initiating the act, and finally that which was once an arc of liquid glory for which any transom was an easy hurdle becomes a pathetic intermittent dribbling that yields more nostalgia than results. This relative obstruction to the flow produces permanent distention of the bladder, which now fails to empty itself entirely.

There results a pool of residual urine, a perfect culture medium for any bacteria wandering by. This combination of obstruction, stagnation and infection sets the stage for the formation of stones in the bladder. Indeed, prior to the advent of modern prostatic surgery, the incidence of bladder stones in men was as common as gallstones are now in women in this age of blintzes and quiche Lorraine.

Although this serves to explain the formation of stones in the bladder, no such etiological rationale exists for the presence of stones in the kidney, where they are today at least as common. Like some mysterious and malicious possession, the plague of kidney stone continues to defy our understanding. Is it due solely to the presence of an excess of one of the salts, such as calcium or magnesium phosphate or uric acid? Is it due to some unknown dietary or vitamin deficiency? An inadequate intake of water which leaves us relatively dehydrated? Or an antecedent abnormality of the tissues of the kidney itself?

A less scientific, more fatalistic approach would be to invoke a *true-grit* theory, that the longer we live the more we tend to harden: first to calcify, then to ossify, and finally, like forests and the plants of the sea, to petrify. One might picture all of history as the slow migration of the human species from one Stone Age to another. Nature does seem to have a way of marbling us in for the long haul.

What risks the urinary system takes!—paying for the fragile beauty of its structure by daring obstruction at any of a number of its tapered straits, either at the entrance of the kidney into the ureter, at the slender junction of the ureter and bladder, or along the path of the male urethra, where, on either side, loom the terrible lobes of the prostate gland. Not Jason and the Argonauts in their passage between the crushing Symplegades, nor Ulysses at the Bosporus, pursued by the ill-tempered malignant Wandering Rocks, surpassed in their voyages the hazards of the urinary flow through the narrows of the prostatic urethra.

That these two men spent altogether too much time skimming across the wine-dark sea for the good of their kidneys is quite apparent. Nor is it beyond the scope of reasonable conjecture that the elderly authors of these two epics, Homer and whoever, themselves suffered from urinary obstruction at this vulnerable site, their art then being but a metaphor of their distress. But since when, one might ask, has it been any different?

What is very real, however, is the agony produced by the stones of the body, for it is generally agreed that there is no pain more severe than that caused by Stone.

Into this idyllic landscape of bowls and strings is born the seed of its destruction. Not smuggled in from without, nor from a rival organ dispatched, but organizing, bunching, salting out from its own tissues, growing massy, a stone is formed, like an inexorable truth.

What is man, the son of man, asks the biochemist, but a container of salt solution in a state of more or less saturation? Ever so slowly he settles out, clouding milkily up, depositing within himself silt, a silt whipped by the slowest of currents and inner winds into serrated banks and whorls. Who knows at what point the balance between solution and precipitation will have been tipped, and the first speck of mineral will appear like the birth of a planet in the void, realizing out of tissues overcharged with calcium, uric acid or others of the stone-forming elements, a mote, a jot, unbeknownst, uncelebrated? No tocsin is sounded, no alarum. Yet toxin and alarm are its business credentials. When is it that the acidity or alkalinity of the urine is so mysteriously altered, and with such a misdirected hospitality, as to encourage the persistence of the wicked speck? Too small by many months, even years, to be seen or felt, it is most importantly THERE, either lodged in some damp cul-de-sac, or carried by hidden currents, crashing against secret membranes, all the while gathering unto itself from the high urinary waters, full as briny as the Dead Sea, more and more of the bitterest crystals, growing slow as diamond, and as cursed, worn only at the greatest risk.

Thus is agony born. The speck hardens, concretes, is overlaid with more salt dust, becomes compressed. Spikes extend from it, pits are excavated, until it has a shape as distinctive as a face. And just as a face widens, elongates, wrinkles, so does the stone. Not warts but stalagmites encrust its surface; not creases, but limy fissures break across it. There in the dank and humid corners of the kidney, the dragony thing lurks until weaned from its cache by the horrid principles of physics and chemistry; or kicked loose by a mocking fate, it slips into the wash of the tubules, abutting against the narrows, pushed by a hydrostatic pressure that knows no turning back.

Then there is Pain. But such a pain as defies the words of mouth or pen to set it down, pain that, by its intensity, elects the sufferer to an aristocracy of endurance, a priesthood of experience, from which all mere mortals are excluded. He who has not felt the bolting gripe of colic in back or side or belly has not the language of this elite, is illiterate of their tongue.

Whom the stone grips is transformed in one instant from man to shark; and like the shark that must remain in perpetual motion, fins and tail moving restlessly lest it, helpless, sink to terrible black depths of pressure, so the harborer of stone writhes and twists, bending and unbending in ceaseless turmoil. Now he straightens, stretches his limbs, only to draw them upon his trunk the next moment and fling his body from one side to another, finding ease in neither. From between his teeth come sounds so primitive and elemental as to trigger the skin to rise and creep. He shudders and vomits, as though to cast forth the rock that grinds within. He would sell his birthright, forfeit his honor, his name, even kill, to rid him of it. He toils in the bed, pronged and spiked from within. Sweat breaks upon his face like seed pearls. In a moment his hair is heavy with

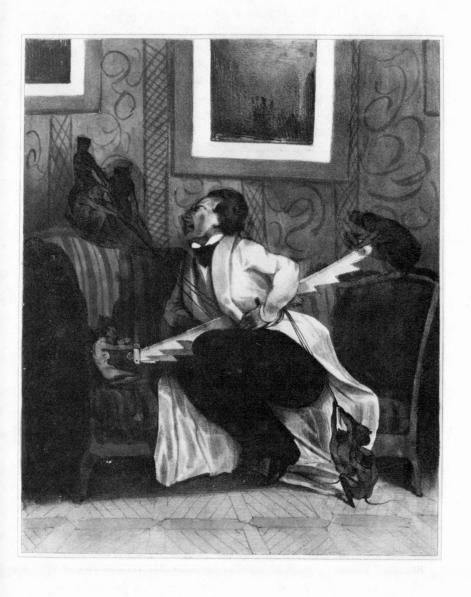

it. The fingers scrabble against the bed, the wall, his own flesh, as if to tear release from these surfaces.

But it does not pass. The impacted stone cannot push through into the lake, or be voided into the open sea. Like some terrible work of art, insatiable, demanding, it screams to be extruded, let out into the air and light, to be seen, touched, venerated, tearing apart its creator, destroying him in the act of deliverance.

At last he is able to force a few drops of bloody urine, and the pain subsides. The stone has fallen away from its point of impaction, washed loose into the bladder. He is miraculously free of pain for a moment. It is no less than being touched by the hand of God. Still, he is afraid to move, desperate lest the slightest change of position should sink the craggy thing again into some new part and the hell be reenacted. It has not passed. It lies within him yet, malevolent, scorpioid. It is only a matter of time before the beast will rise to feed again.

Such is the purity, the unclouded nature of the pain of stone as to have welded its sufferers into a fellowship magnificent in its perfection. It is curious that no pleasure, no joy, nor even any ecstasy, either sexual or religious, has the power to produce such a deathless amalgamation of the spirit among human beings. It is only pain, especially the pain of the stone, that is the catalyst, the beating heart of such high possibility.

Indeed, the fraternity of pain includes a great number of men of quality. Montaigne, the French essayist, writes: "I feel everywhere Men tormented with the same Disease: and am honour'd by the Fellowship, forasmuch as Men of the best Quality are most frequently afflicted with it; 'tis a noble and dignified Disease. And were it not a good office to a man to put him in mind of his end? My kidneys claw me to purpose."

Of those lettered men who have at one time or another

felt the terrible gripe of the stone, it must be conceded that Montaigne was the emblem, the grand seigneur. Of the others, Cicero was the luckiest, reporting, as he did, to have discharged his stone in the sheets while dreaming he lay with a wench. What a pity Montaigne had not the faculties of that Roman wet-dreamer.

Nevertheless, Montaigne insisted upon the bright side. He compared the relief he felt after voiding a stone to that of Socrates enjoying the scratching of the itch made by his chains immediately after they were removed. Unlike many other illnesses that are years in recovering, and leave residual distempers aplenty, the passed stone carries itself clean off. Too, the suffering is so great that it purifies, purges the body of other ill humors. "It is a physick in itself for absolute deliverance." Stone plays its game by itself, lets Montaigne play his. One has only to endure. Nothing one does can relieve it or make it worse. Play, run, ride, debauch. It will affect you neither for good nor ill. Say as much, if you can, for the pox, the gout, or bursten belly. Other diseases rack all our actions, disturb our whole order; this only pinches the skin, leaves the understanding and will at our disposal, as also the tongue and the hands and feet. It rather awakes than stupefies you. "The stone does not meddle with the soul." Four centuries later, V. S. Pritchett was to put it more colloquially, when his blind man says, "So long as you've got your legs you can give yourself an airing."

Rationalizations, you say. Perhaps, but divine ones that enabled not only Montaigne to live, but generations of his descendants as well. No man lives that has ever felt the gripe and point of stone who does not love Montaigne.

Samuel Pepys, who first felt the symptoms of his stone while a student at Cambridge, dared the rigors of unanesthetized surgery and lived, cured, to exhibit his prize, the size of a tennis ball, in an elaborate wooden reliquary carved for this purpose. Even now it pains me to envision the little man with the great heart held to the edge of a table by four strong restrainers, while the dreaded surgeon Hollier plunged the knife into his perineum, cleaving directly into the bladder and drawing forth the huge rock. Each year thereafter, on the anniversary of his deliverance, Pepys held a party for all his friends, and fellow sufferers, at which fetes the various calculi were passed hand to hand, like saintly relics, and venerated by the guests. The diary entry for March 26, 1662, on the fourth anniversary of his cutting for stone: "Up early, this being by God's great blessing the fourth solemn day of my cutting for the stone. At noon came my good guests. I had a pretty dinner for them—a brace of stewed carps, six roasted chickens, and a jowl of salmon hot, followed by a tansy, two neats' tongues and cheese. We were very merry all the afternoon, talking and singing and piping upon the flageolette." Pepys's surgeon, Hollier, cut thirty-four stone in one year, and all lived, and afterward cut four and all died. Fortunate for Pepys that he was operated upon before Hollier's instruments became septic. For other more aristocratic such gatherings, English and French dandies caused cards to be made, beautiful cards, each bearing a picture of their stone and the date of their operation.

A far cry indeed from the unrhapsodized hosts of the stoned of Asia. It was ever thus. In India and Thailand, it is particularly the children who suffer from stone, in some areas the condition being all but universal. It is thought to owe to the custom of women to premasticate their infants' food, chewing up the mash, mixing it with their own saliva before spitting it, birdlike, directly into the mouths of their young. It is a mess quite devoid of the essential amino acids necessary for proper metabolism of calcium in the body. This calcium then, roiling grittily through the bloodstream in great concentrations, is filtered out into the kidneys and finds its way into the tiny bladder, where begins the insidious, ineluctable growth that leads to either the agony of surgery or death. In one village in northwest Thailand there is a street that is paved with the bladder stones of its children. Such a path would scald the feet of Genghis Khan. The lingering cries of the children must creep up the legs, paralyzing any who would walk this via dolorosa.

In 1739, a woman named Joanna Stephens was paid five thousand pounds by the British government for the secret composition of her stone solvent. It was promptly published in the *London Gazette* and read by another sufferer, Horace Walpole, who with his brother swilled great quantities of the stuff and swore it cured them of their stones. The recipe was a mixture of eggshells, snails and soap. Obsessed by the subject of stone, Walpole, in one of his letters, reported of a certain Archbishop Stone, "The Primate wears in a ring the stone Lady Northumberland voided in Dublin." Further, he gossiped, the Lady Mary Wortley said: "People wish their enemies dead—but I do not; I say give them gout, give them the stone." David Garrick, the most famous actor of Walpole's day, had the stone *and* gout. Despite this, he nightly danced a country dance in Benjamin Hoadly's comedy *The Suspicious Husband*. Walpole attended and envied, not his performance, but his physical capabilities.

Benjamin Franklin was still another victim, a sort of unlucky Pierre. Above all others, he appears to have taken Montaigne's advice to heart, not permitting his ailment to interfere with his livelier activities. Whether it was in compensation for his stones or to spite them, he succeeded in being our most Parisian ambassador to France, thereby calling upon his hosts to put their money where their mouths were in the matter of debauchery. The noble Franklin nevertheless endured his rigors in private, often having to stand on his head to void when his bladder stone fell into the urethral opening and blocked it off. He discovered that in this position he could dislodge the rock and empty his bladder. With characteristic ingenuity, Franklin invented a better catheter, which he used so successfully upon himself to draw his water that he had another one made and sent to his brother who also suffered from the stone. Franklin placed this contribution far above the mere harnessing of electricity or the publication of an ordinary almanac.

Why dwell on the sufferings of those long gone? To what purpose? True it is that we cannot bear our lives, our work, our pain without the companionship of the past. It helps the deaf man to know that Beethoven could not hear his own glory, the blind that Milton too dwelt in darkness. That Keats and Chopin endured the fevers and the bloody cough of tuberculosis is balm in Gilead to those more recently afflicted. What disenfranchised homosexual cannot take comfort in the imprisonment of Oscar Wilde in Reading Gaol?

Suffering is the bond that transcends time and place, the barriers of language and race. It is to the *heritage* of our private affliction that we turn in moments of direst stress. From it we draw the courage to bear whatever it is that has been thrust upon us. So it is with the fellowship of the stone. The same craggy rocks that pronged the vitals of Montaigne scrape the membranes of the twentieth-century bladder.

What is history for, if not to offer aid and comfort to the living? Not to draw upon it is to be like the beasts who feel the full pain of their wounds without recourse to the narcosis of the past. Thus did Montaigne, ground toward the edge by the pain of his stone, writing *against* the pain, gaze back at the ancients of Greece and Rome, in envy and admiration, and finally in fraternity.

The surgery for the removal of bladder stones is among the oldest in the history of medicine. Reported in the ancient Sumerian literature, and again during the Pharaonic dynasties of Egypt, lithotomy, or cutting for stone, reached its highest form in seventeenth- and eighteenth-century France and England. This despite the fact that Hippocrates in his oath, still taken by every graduating medical student, specifically forbids both abortion and cutting for stone.

The most famous lithotomist of all time was not a doctor but an itinerant thug named Jacques Baulot, whose medical career began in 1680 as servant to Pauloni, a strolling lithotomist and curer of ruptures. It was Baulot's task to restrain the patients during surgery. With a rugged individualism more natural to Elmer Gantry than to, say, Harvey Cushing, this worthy decided that he could do it better himself, and that he'd certainly much rather. Donning the religious habit of a monk of the order of Saint Francis, but affecting also a huge, black, broad-brimmed hat, Baulot called himself Frère Jacques and traveled about Italy and France cutting the stone out of anyone who would lie still long enough. Soon the word of his extraordinary dexterity had spread, and by the end of the seventeenth century, Baulot was a familiar figure at any number of the royal courts of Europe, as lithotomist to kings. In fact, he *was* better than anyone else, and thoroughly deserving of the wine, women, and song rained upon him by grateful princes.

It is not, I assure you, sour surgical grapes that prompt me to remark that not a little of Baulot's success was due to his costume. It is true that we have lost the art of dressing up to look the part of our profession, and it is regrettable that one can no longer distinguish between surgeons and musicians in the park. Personally, I have always envied Frère Jacques his habit and his hat.

Today's urologists are a deft but underdressed lot to whom lithotomy and prostatectomy are an easy jug of jam, and who do not hesitate to make free use of catheter and cystoscope despite the justifiable notion among the public that such are the instruments of ultimate violation.

And what of the future?

There is reason for hope.

Stones are today being dissolved with special solvents taken as medication. Ultrasonic waves directed into the hollow organs of dogs are capable of shattering some stones into solution. Both methods are still considered experimental and outside the realm of practicability for general medicine. Perhaps one day soon we shall be rid of our stones by one or another of these methods. Good riddance, we shall say, as with all diseases that are made curable.

Still, I shall always see the story of the stone as a kind of alchemy in which common minerals were transformed into golden truth.

THE KNIFE

One holds the knife as one holds the bow of a cello or a tulip—by the stem. Not palmed nor gripped nor grasped, but lightly, with the tips of the fingers. The knife is not for pressing. It is for drawing across the field of skin. Like a slender fish, it waits, at the ready, then, go! It darts, followed by a fine wake of red. The flesh parts, falling away to yellow globules of fat. Even now, after so many times, I still marvel at its power—cold, gleaming, silent. More, I am still struck with a kind of dread that it is I in whose hand the blade travels, that my hand is its vehicle, that yet again this terrible steel-bellied thing and I have conspired for a most unnatural purpose, the laying open of the body of a human being.

A stillness settles in my heart and is carried to my hand. It is the quietude of resolve layered over fear. And it is this resolve that lowers us, my knife and me, deeper and deeper into the person beneath. It is an entry into the body that is nothing like a caress; still, it is among the gentlest of acts. Then stroke and stroke again, and we are joined by other instruments, hemostats and forceps, until the wound blooms with strange flowers whose looped handles fall to the sides in steely array.

There is sound, the tight click of clamps fixing teeth into

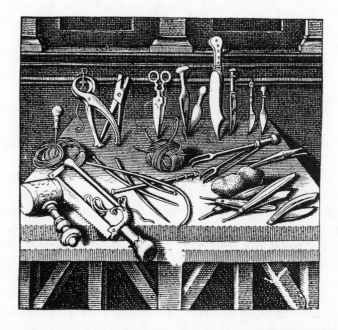

severed blood vessels, the snuffle and gargle of the suction machine clearing the field of blood for the next stroke, the litany of monosyllables with which one prays his way down and in: *clamp, sponge, suture, tie, cut.* And there is color. The green of the cloth, the white of the sponges, the red and yellow of the body. Beneath the fat lies the fascia, the tough fibrous sheet encasing the muscles. It must be sliced and the red beef of the muscles separated. Now there are retractors to hold apart the wound. Hands move together, part, weave. We are fully engaged, like children absorbed in a game or the craftsmen of some place like Damascus.

Deeper still. The peritoneum, pink and gleaming and membranous, bulges into the wound. It is grasped with forceps, and opened. For the first time we can see into the cavity of the abdomen. Such a primitive place. One expects to find drawings of buffalo on the walls. The sense of trespassing is keener now, heightened by the world's light illuminating the organs, their secret colors revealed—maroon and salmon and yellow. The vista is sweetly vulnerable at this moment, a kind of welcoming. An arc of the liver shines high and on the right, like a dark sun. It laps over the pink sweep of the stomach, from whose lower border the gauzy omentum is draped, and through which veil one sees, sinuous, slow as just-fed snakes, the indolent coils of the intestine.

You turn aside to wash your gloves. It is a ritual cleansing. One enters this temple doubly washed. Here is man as microcosm, representing in all his parts the earth, perhaps the universe.

I must confess that the priestliness of my profession has ever been impressed on me. In the beginning there are vows, taken with all solemnity. Then there is the endless harsh novitiate of training, much fatigue, much sacrifice. At last one emerges as celebrant, standing close to the truth lying curtained in the Ark of the body. Not surplice and cassock but mask and gown are your regalia. You hold no chalice, but a knife. There is no wine, no wafer. There are only the facts of blood and flesh.

And if the surgeon is like a poet, then the scars you have made on countless bodies are like verses into the fashioning of which you have poured your soul. I think that if years later I were to see the trace from an old incision of mine, I should know it at once, as one recognizes his pet expressions.

But mostly you are a traveler in a dangerous country, advancing into the moist and jungly cleft your hands have made. Eyes and ears are shuttered from the land you left behind; mind empties itself of all other thought. You are the root of groping fingers. It is a fine hour for the fingers, their sense of touch so enhanced. The blind must know this feeling. Oh, there is risk everywhere. One goes lightly. The spleen. No! No! Do not touch the spleen that lurks below the left leaf of the diaphragm, a manta ray in a coral cave, its bloody tongue protruding. One poke and it might rupture, exploding with sudden hemorrhage. The filmy omentum must not be torn, the intestine scraped or denuded. The hand finds the liver, palms it, fingers running along its sharp lower edge, admiring. Here are the twin mounds of the kidneys, the apron of the omentum hanging in front of the intestinal coils. One lifts it aside and the fingers dip among the loops, searching, mapping territory, establishing boundaries. Deeper still, and the womb is touched, then held like a small muscular bottle—the womb and its earlike appendages, the ovaries. How they do nestle in the cup of a man's hand, their power all dormant. They are frailty itself.

There is a hush in the room. Speech stops. The hands of the others, assistants and nurses, are still. Only the voice of the patient's respiration remains. It is the rhythm of a quiet sea, the sound of waiting. Then you speak, slowly, the terse entries of a Himalayan climber reporting back.

"The stomach is okay. Greater curvature clean. No sign of ulcer. Pylorus, duodenum fine. Now comes the gallbladder. No stones. Right kidney, left, all right. Liver . . . uh-oh."

Your speech lowers to a whisper, falters, stops for a long, long moment, then picks up again at the end of a sigh that comes through your mask like a last exhalation.

"Three big hard ones in the left lobe, one on the right. Metastatic deposits. Bad, bad. Where's the primary? Got to be coming from somewhere."

The arm shifts direction and the fingers drop lower and lower into the pelvis—the body impaled now upon the arm of the surgeon to the hilt of the elbow.

"Here it is."

The voice goes flat, all business now.

"Tumor in the sigmoid colon, wrapped all around it,

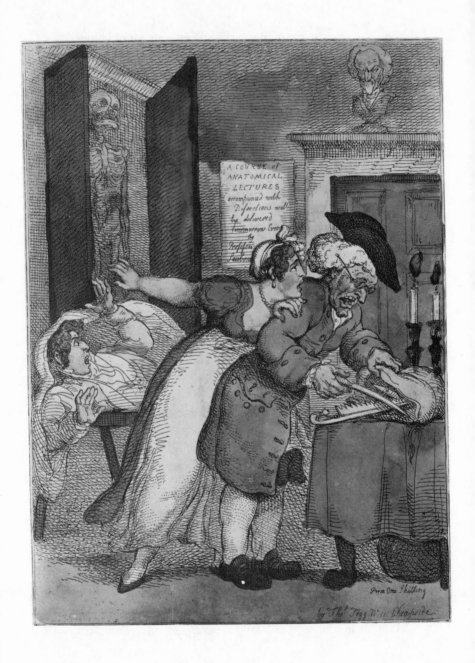

A COURSE of
ANATOMICAL
LECTURES
accompanied with
Dissections will
be delivered
tomorrow Even.g
by
Professor
Lectures

Price One Shilling

by Tho.s Tegg N.o 111 Cheapside.

pretty tight. We'll take out a sleeve of the bowel. No co-
lostomy. Not that, anyway. But, God, there's a lot of it
down there. Here, you take a feel."

You step back from the table, and lean into a sterile basin
of water, resting on stiff arms, while the others locate the
cancer.

When I was a small boy, I was taken by my father, a
general practitioner in Troy, New York, to St. Mary's
Hospital, to wait while he made his rounds. The solarium
where I sat was all sunlight and large plants. It smelled of
soap and starch and clean linen. In the spring, clouds of
lilac billowed from the vases; and in the fall, chrysanthe-
mums crowded the magazine tables. At one end of the
great high-ceilinged, glass-walled room was a huge cage
where colored finches streaked and sang. Even from the
first, I sensed the nearness of that other place, the Operating Room, knew that somewhere on these premises was
that secret dreadful enclosure where *surgery* was at that
moment happening. I sat among the cut flowers, half drunk
on the scent, listening to the robes of the nuns brush the
walls of the corridor, and felt the awful presence of *surgery*.

Oh, the pageantry! I longed to go there. I feared to go
there. I imagined surgeons bent like storks over the body of
the patient, a circle of red painted across the abdomen.
Silence and dignity and awe enveloped them, these surgeons; it was the bubble in which they bent and straightened. Ah, it was a place I would never see, a place from
whose walls the hung and suffering Christ turned his affliction to highest purpose. It is thirty years since I yearned for
that old Surgery. And now I merely break the beam of an
electric eye, and double doors swing open to let me enter,
and as I enter, always, I feel the surging of a force that I
feel in no other place. It is as though I am suddenly
stronger and larger, heroic. Yes, that's it!

The operating room is called a theatre. One walks onto a set where the cupboards hold tanks of oxygen and other gases. The cabinets store steel cutlery of unimagined versatility, and the refrigerators are filled with bags of blood. Bodies are stroked and penetrated here, but no love is made. Nor is it ever allowed to grow dark, but must always gleam with a grotesque brightness. For the special congress into which patient and surgeon enter, the one must have his senses deadened, the other his sensibilities restrained. One lies naked, blind, offering; the other stands masked and gloved. One yields; the other does his will.

I said no love is made here, but love happens. I have stood aside with lowered gaze while a priest, wearing the purple scarf of office, administers Last Rites to the man I shall operate upon. I try not to listen to those terrible last questions, the answers, but hear, with scorching clarity, the words that formalize the expectation of death. For a moment my resolve falters before the resignation, the *attentiveness*, of the other two. I am like an executioner who hears the cleric comforting the prisoner. For the moment I am excluded from the centrality of the event, a mere technician standing by. But it is only for the moment.

The priest leaves, and we are ready. Let it begin.

Later, I am repairing the strangulated hernia of an old man. Because of his age and frailty, I am using local anesthesia. He is awake. His name is Abe Kaufman, and he is a Russian Jew. A nurse sits by his head, murmuring to him. She wipes his forehead. I know her very well. Her name is Alexandria, and she is the daughter of Ukrainian peasants. She has a flat steppe of a face and slanting eyes. Nurse and patient are speaking of blintzes, borscht, piroshki—Russian food that they both love. I listen, and think that it may have been her grandfather who raided the shtetl where the old man lived long ago, and in his high boots and his blouse and his fury this grandfather pulled Abe by his side curls to the ground and stomped his face and kicked his groin. Perhaps it was that ancient kick that caused the hernia I am fixing. I listen to them whispering behind the screen at the head of the table. I listen with breath held before the prism of history.

"Tovarich," she says, her head bent close to his.

He smiles up at her, and forgets that his body is being laid open.

"You are an angel," the old man says.

One can count on absurdity. There, in the midst of our solemnities, appears, small and black and crawling, an insect: The Ant of the Absurd. The belly is open; one has seen and felt the catastrophe within. It seems the patient is already vaporizing into angelhood in the heat escaping therefrom. One could warm one's hands in that fever. All at once that ant is there, emerging from beneath one of the sterile towels that border the operating field. For a moment one does not really see it, or else denies the sight, so impossible it is, marching precisely, heading briskly toward the open wound.

Drawn from its linen lair, where it snuggled in the steam of the great sterilizer, and survived, it comes. Closer and closer, it hurries toward the incision. Ant, art thou in the grip of some fatal *ivresse?* Wouldst hurtle over these scarlet cliffs into the very boil of the guts? Art mad for the reek we handle? Or in some secret act of formication engaged?

The alarm is sounded. An ant! An ant! And we are unnerved. Our fear of defilement is near to frenzy. It is not the mere physical contamination that we loathe. It is the evil of the interloper, that he scurries across our holy place, and filthies our altar. He *is* disease—that for whose destruction we have gathered. Powerless to destroy the sickness before us, we turn to its incarnation with a vengeance, and pluck it from the lip of the incision in the nick of time. Who would have thought an ant could move so fast?

Between thumb and forefinger, the intruder is crushed.
It dies as quietly as it lived. Ah, but now there is death in
the room. It is a perversion of our purpose. Albert Schweit-
zer would have spared it, scooped it tenderly into his hand,
and lowered it to the ground.

The corpselet is flicked into the specimen basin. The
gloves are changed. New towels and sheets are placed
where it walked. We are pleased to have done something, if
only a small killing. The operation resumes, and we draw
upon ourselves once more the sleeves of office and rank. Is
our reverence for life in question?

In the room the instruments lie on trays and tables. They
are arranged precisely by the scrub nurse, in an order that
never changes, so that you can reach blindly for a forceps
or hemostat without looking away from the operating
field. The instruments lie *thus!* Even at the beginning,
when all is clean and tidy and no blood has been spilled, it is
the scalpel that dominates. It has a figure the others do not
have, the retractors and the scissors. The scalpel is all grace
and line, a fierceness. It grins. It is like a cat—to be re-
spected, deferred to, but which returns no amiability. To
hold it above a belly is to know the knife's force—as
though were you to give it slightest rein, it would pursue
an intent of its own, driving into the flesh, a wild energy.

In a story by Borges, a deadly knife fight between two
rivals is depicted. It is not, however, the men who are fight-
ing. It is the knives themselves that are settling their own
old score. The men who hold the knives are mere adjuncts
to the weapons. The unguarded knife is like the unbridled
war-horse that not only carries its helpless rider to his
death, but tramples all beneath its hooves. The hand of the
surgeon must tame this savage thing. He is a rider reining to
capture a pace.

So close is the joining of knife and surgeon that they are
like the Centaur—the knife, below, all equine energy, the

surgeon, above, with his delicate art. One holds the knife back as much as advances it to purpose. One is master of the scissors. One is partner, sometimes rival, to the knife. In a moment it is like the long red fingernail of the Dragon Lady. Thus does the surgeon curb in order to create, restraining the scalpel, governing it shrewdly, setting the action of the operation into a pattern, giving it form and purpose.

It is the nature of creatures to live within a tight cuirass that is both their constriction and their protection. The carapace of the turtle is his fortress and retreat, yet keeps him writhing on his back in the sand. So is the surgeon rendered impotent by his own empathy and compassion. The surgeon cannot weep. When he cuts the flesh, his own must not bleed. Here it is all work. Like an asthmatic hungering for air, longing to take just one deep breath, the surgeon struggles not to feel. It is suffocating to press the feeling out. It would be easier to weep or mourn—for you know that the lovely precise world of proportion contains, just beneath, *there*, all disaster, all disorder. In a surgical operation, a risk may flash into reality: the patient dies . . . of *complication*. The patient knows this too, in a more direct and personal way, and he is afraid.

And what of that *other*, the patient, you, who are brought to the operating room on a stretcher, having been washed and purged and dressed in a white gown? Fluid drips from a bottle into your arm, diluting you, leaching your body of its personal brine. As you wait in the corridor, you hear from behind the closed door the angry clang of steel upon steel, as though a battle were being waged. There is the odor of antiseptic and ether, and masked women hurry up and down the halls, in and out of rooms. There is the watery sound of strange machinery, the tinny beeping that is the transmitted heartbeat of yet another *human being*. And all the while the dreadful knowledge that soon you will be taken, laid beneath great lamps that will reveal the secret linings of your body. In the very act of lying down, you have made a declaration of surrender. One lies down gladly for sleep or for love. But to give over one's body and will for surgery, to *lie down* for it, is a yielding of more than we can bear.

Soon a man will stand over you, gowned and hooded. In time the man will take up a knife and crack open your flesh like a ripe melon. Fingers will rummage among your viscera. Parts of you will be cut out. Blood will run free. Your blood. All the night before you have turned with the presentiment of death upon you. You have attended your funeral, wept with your mourners. You think, "I should never have had surgery in the springtime." It is too cruel. Or on a Thursday. It is an unlucky day.

Now it is time. You are wheeled in and moved to the table. An injection is given. "Let yourself go," I say. "It's a pleasant sensation," I say. "Give in," I say.

Let go? Give in? When you know that you are being tricked into the hereafter, that you will end when consciousness ends? As the monstrous silence of anesthesia falls discourteously across your brain, you watch your soul drift off.

Later, in the recovery room, you awaken and gaze through the thickness of drugs at the world returning, and you guess, at first dimly, then surely, that you have not died. In pain and nausea you will know the exultation of death averted, of life restored.

What is it, then, this thing, the knife, whose shape is virtually the same as it was three thousand years ago, but now with its head grown detachable? Before steel, it was bronze. Before bronze, stone—then back into unremembered time. Did man invent it or did the knife precede him here, hidden under ages of vegetation and hoofprints, lying in wait to be discovered, picked up, used?

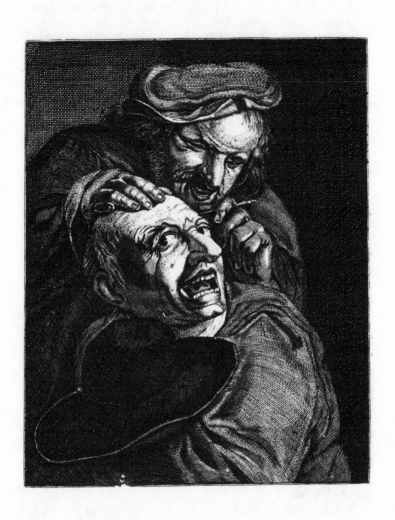

The scalpel is in two parts, the handle and the blade. Joined, it is six inches from tip to tip. At one end of the handle is a narrow notched prong upon which the blade is slid, then snapped into place. Without the blade, the handle has a blind, decapitated look. It is helpless as a trussed maniac. But slide on the blade, click it home, and the knife springs instantly to life. It is headed now, edgy, leaping to mount the fingers for the gallop to its feast.

Now is the moment from which you have turned aside, from which you have averted your gaze, yet toward which you have been hastened. Now the scalpel sings along the flesh again, its brute run unimpeded by germs or other frictions. It is a slick slide home, a barracuda spurt, a rip of embedded talon. One listens, and almost hears the whine—nasal, high, delivered through that gleaming metallic snout. The flesh splits with its own kind of moan. It is like the penetration of rape.

The breasts of women are cut off, arms and legs sliced to the bone to make ready for the saw, eyes freed from sockets, intestines lopped. The hand of the surgeon rebels. Tension boils through his pores, like sweat. The flesh of the patient retaliates with hemorrhage, and the blood chases the knife wherever it is withdrawn.

Within the belly a tumor squats, toadish, fungoid. A gray mother and her brood. The only thing it does not do is croak. It too is hacked from its bed as the carnivore knife lips the blood, turning in it in a kind of ecstasy of plenty, a gluttony after the long fast. It is just for this that the knife was created, tempered, heated, its violence beaten into paper-thin force.

At last a little thread is passed into the wound and tied. The monstrous booming fury is stilled by a tiny thread. The tempest is silenced. The operation is over. On the table, the knife lies spent, on its side, the bloody meal smear-dried upon its flanks. The knife rests.

And waits.

SKIN

I sing of skin, layered fine as baklava, whose colors shame the dawn, at once the scabbard upon which is writ our only signature, and the instrument by which we are thrilled, protected, and kept constant in our natural place. Here is each man bagged and trussed in perfect amiability. See how it upholsters the bone and muscle underneath, now accenting the point of an elbow, now rolling over the pectorals to hollow the grotto of an armpit. Nippled and umbilicated, and perforated by the most diverse and marvelous openings, each with its singular rim and curtain. Thus the carven helix of the ear, the rigid nostrils, the puckered continence of the anus, the moist and sensitive lips of mouth and vagina.

What is it, then, this seamless body-stocking, some two yards square, this our casing, our façade, that flushes, pales, perspires, glistens, glows, furrows, tingles, crawls, itches, pleasures, and pains us all our days, at once keeper of the organs within, and sensitive probe, adventurer into the world outside?

Come, let us explore: there exists the rosy coast, these estuaries of pearl.

Gaze upon the skin as I have, through a microscope brightly, and tremble at the wisdom of God, for here is a magic tissue to suit all seasons. Two layers compose the skin—the superficial epidermis and, deeper, the dermis. Between is a plane of pure energy where the life-force is in full gallop. Identical cells spring full-grown here, each as tall and columnar as its brother, to form an unbroken line over the body. No sooner are these cells formed than they move toward the surface, whether drawn to the open air by some protoplasmic hunger or pushed outward by the birth of still newer cells behind. In migration the skin cells flatten, first to cubes, then plates. Twenty-six days later the plates are no more than attenuated wisps of keratin meshed together to guard against forces that would damage the skin by shearing or compression. Here they lie, having lost all semblance of living cellularity, until they are shed from the body in a continuous dismal rain. Thus into the valley of death this number marches in well-stepped soldiery, gallant, summoned to a sacrifice beyond its ken. But . . . let the skin be cut or burned, and the brigade breaks into a charge, fanning out laterally across the wound, racing to seal off the defect. The margins are shored up; healing earthworks are raised, and guerrilla squads of invading bacteria are isolated and mopped up. The reserves too are called to the colors and the rate of mitosis increases throughout the injured area. Hurrah for stratified squamous epithelium!

Beneath the epidermis lies the dermis, a resilient pad of elastic tissue in which glands, hair follicles, nerves and blood vessels are arranged in infinitely variable mosaic. Within this rich bed three million sweat glands lie; these, in full sluice, can extract from the blood up to three kilograms of fluid in a single hour. Such a warm fall cools the body even as it evaporates from its surface and, incidentally, flushes from us the excess of salt that threatens to make of the body juices a pickling brine. In this, the sweat glands are helpmates to the kidney. Ah, but the skin *harbors* water and heat as well, containing our fluid and blood lest, one sunny day, we leak our way to dusty desiccation on some pavement or, bitten, bleed an hour or two, and die.

These sweat glands are most numerous on the palms and soles, and have their highest density at birth, decreasing steadily thereafter. Only the glans penis, clitoris, labia minora, and the inner surface of the prepuce have no sweat glands, a curiously sexual deficiency that ought to tell us something, but for God's sake what?

Never mind. Exclusiveness, in no matter what context, is not without its charms.

Still other glands of the dermis yield odoriferous oils. In that they attract mates and repel enemies, these musky syrups, called pheromones, engage in a kind of cutaneous communication. One may well deplore the perverse vanity which insists that we spray, roll on, and dab our flesh sobs to deny these darling chemicals their true role. To banish our natural stink is to play havoc with no less than the procreative process itself, depriving it of its olfactory joys, at the very least. Such misguided fastidiousness will do us no good in the end. Keep in mind, a single sniff of phero- mone can raise expectations to which a whole Pacific of perfume cannot pretend, nor an Atlantic of attar attain.

Besides, some of us need all the help we can get.

Ranking with the earlobes as our most adorable gewgaws are the nails that decorate the fingers and toes. One parts with the nails only under political duress and in great pain. Long since having retired their acquisitive and protective functions, they are more like the sweet hooflets of a year- ling than the talons of a hawk. Still, among guitar players, certain Japanese weavers, and women with time on their hands, length is prized. For such specialists as for all who find it impossible to go on without knowing, it must be put abroad that nails grow faster in the dominant hand, grow twenty percent faster in the summer than in the winter, and grow twice as fast during the day as at night. Pregnancy, trauma, and nail-biting (mother's bane) are said to increase the rate of nail growth.

Four living paints, called biochromes, combine to give the skin its color at any given moment. There are brown, yellow, bright red, and purplish red. The bright red is called oxyhemoglobin and is carried by the blood to the skin. In the state of anemia or hemorrhage, there is less blood, thus less bright red, and the skin whitens, turns pale, until the line between pillowcase and patient is as indistinct as any horizon where sea and sky blend. Among those so afflicted were Elizabeth Barrett Browning, Annabel Lee, and The Lady of the Camellias. It is all very nineteenth-century.

Melanin is the brown pigment, which, under the influence of glands afar, gives to the skin what darkness it has. Without it we are albinos—pink, wretched creatures whose oxyhemoglobin is not masked by melanin, and for whom the sun's rays are no solace but ten thousand cruel fires that anger and abrade the tissues to malignancy.

It is differences in the number and size of pigment granules called melanosomes that account for whether your skin is naturally black or white. If your skin is black, you own more and larger of these organelles. But it happens that, for as yet unexplained reasons, a man may turn piebald.

Think, if you will, upon one Henry Moss. In Goochland County, Virginia, sprang he, black as an eggplant, from the loins of his mother and father in the otherwise unremembered year of 1754. Farmers his begetters were, and so did young Henry remain until the Revolutionary War broke out. He was twenty-two, and with many other free blacks, he enlisted in the Colonial Army, where he served for six

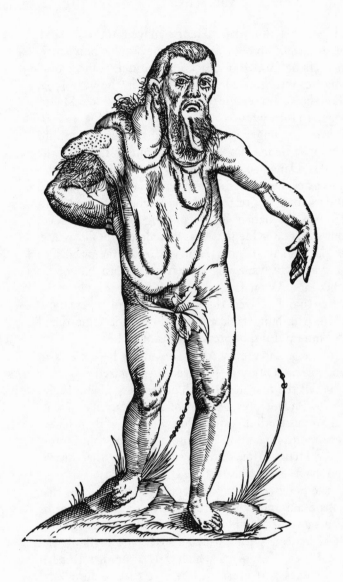

years. Upon his discharge, Henry moved to Maryland, married, and took up once again his hoe and his plowshare. For ten years he farmed in peaceful anonymity, and would have done so until he died, had not Fate, in the year 1792, given him her most enigmatic smile—for in 1792 Henry Moss began to turn white.

First from his fingertips did the rich blackness fade—to no mere cocoa or tan, but to such a white as matched the fairness of a Dane. Soon the snowy tide had flooded his wrists, his arms, his neck. Next, his chest and abdomen and back undarkened in great irregular patches. He was Holstein. He was Dalmatian. The blanching spread, coalesced, until four years later Henry Moss was almost totally white. Imagine the dismay of poor Henry Moss as he gazed into his mirror and saw vanishing therefrom the last bits of his dermal heritage. What face was this, what head, where the once kinky wool crisped thick and full, and where now limp white hair hung lank and silky? Was it some dread leprosy? Some awful spot presaging dissolution?

Not for long was Henry Moss to wander his little farm alone and palely loitering, for even as he gazed into that mirror, he felt the first fierce fetch of fame . . . and Philadelphia! To Philadelphia, Athens of America, city of culture and sophistication, came Henry Moss with his new whiteness upon him, and in his bosom the glory that transfigures, for Henry Moss had gazed deep into that mirror and seen reflected there his fortune and his destiny.

It was the practice of the innkeepers and hostelers of that time to maintain upon their premises for the enjoyment of their clients any of a number of oddities of natural history. There was a dead whale which had been caught in the Delaware River; a pygarg, which was a strange Russian beast, part camel, part bear; a learned pig that could tell the time of day and who transmitted this data in cunning little grunts; and Miss Sarah Rogers, who, born without arms or legs, still managed to paint elegant flowers and to thread needles with her lips and tongue and teeth. To these was added Henry Moss, the black man who was turning white! Scrub him hard, and see for yourself.

Overnight Henry Moss became a star. For his appearance at Mr. Leech's tavern on Market Street, The Sign of the Black Horse, handbills were passed out upon the streets. A GREAT CURIOSITY, the handbills proclaimed, a sight to open "a wide field of amusement for the philosophical genius."

But Henry Moss was no mere odd outscouring of the human race, suitable only for gawking. Henry Moss wore a message that rocked the very roofbeams of racial chauvinism so muscularly buttressed by our forefathers. Henry Moss was proof that the races were interchangeable, the skin reversible. As naught now, the vaunted difference. Black was white. Why not white . . . black? Why not, indeed!

In time Henry Moss was brought before a convocation of the leading physicians of Philadelphia, where the matter was discussed. Questions were raised, debates joined. Was the source of blackness to be found in the peculiar climate of Africa? If uprooted for a generation or two, would the black essence recede, to be replaced by the white? Would Henry Moss reblacken if transported to Africa? Would the progeny of a white turn black over there? Or was it indeed some perverse chemistry of the skin?

No answers were given. And the celebrated case of Henry Moss faded as swiftly as had the color of his skin. Still, one is left to wonder. . . . Had the good doctors of Philadelphia been led to believe in the interchangeability of the races, might not the blot of slavery, the Civil War itself, have been overleaped? Do you think Henry's *vitiglio* (a disease in which the pigment cells mysteriously fail to produce melanin) might have changed the course of history? Well, it didn't.

And what of Henry Moss? He surfaced last in rural

Georgia where he earned a modest keep showing himself in the saloons of that back country. Like many a fading star, Henry ended playing the boonies.

The skin is the screen upon which the state of the other organs is cast. One can read their health in its condition and hue.

Ails the liver? Then the skin yellows into jaundice as the dislocated bile floods across it.

In the anemic state, the skin turns paper white as the enfeebled blood fails, until it would seem that a mere blush would divert blood enough to send the body into shock.

The first sign of certain cancers hidden deep within the body is itching of the skin or a painful rash.

Trouble in the brain is often heralded by the disappearance of feeling in a part of the skin.

In the poverty of oxygen lack, the skin leadens, is prinked with purple.

So it goes, as the skin reflects the occult mishaps of the marshy interior. It is upon the skin that the calamities of the flesh are made most brutally apparent. Here is all decay realized, all blight and blister exposed.

Awed and hurting, the diabetic watches his feet advance from bevelled grace through sore and ulcer to the blunt black scab of gangrene, extrapolating, as he must, from the part to the sum of his parts, to the whole, and feeling for his sad sweet blood only the most anguished rue.

The youth whose face blazes with rubies and carbuncles would sell his birthright, mortgage his future, to peel his soiled mask from him and don another. But there is no other. Nor any acnesarium where he might hide his pimentoes, eschewing both the pleasures and the risks of new manhood. He is badly touched indeed.

And what heartbroken psoriatic, surveying his embattled skin, would not volunteer for an unanesthetized flaying could it but rid him of his pink sequins, his silver spangles?

I hold no brief for rosy, turgid youth. It does but stir envy and leave compassion unaroused. My sympathies lie with the aging—those, motley with spots, gypsy with plaques and knobs, in whom each misfeatured stain announces with grim certainty the relentless slouching toward . . . the end. Those in whom the elastica has so "given" that one is hung with dewlaps and is with wrinkled crepe empanoplied, in whom neither surgery, nor paints, nor other borrowed trumpery can anymore dissemble, they are the creatures that my heart and my feelings are tied to—those whose state of grace is marginal, the ragtail and bobtag, those in whom the difference from homely to comely is but a single freckle, one wart, a crease.

Yes, my sympathies lie with *us*.

Imagine God as tailor. His shelves are lined with rolls of skin, each with its subtleties of texture and hue. Six days a week He cuts lengths with which to wrap those small piles of flesh and bone into the clever parcels we call babies. Now engage the irreverence to consider that, either out of the tedium born of infinity, or out of mere sly parsimony, He uses for the occasional handicraft a remnant of yard goods, the last of an otherwise perfect bolt, dusty, soiled, perhaps a bit too small or large, one whose woof is warped or that is cut on the bias. I have received many such people in my examination rooms. Like imperfect postage stamps, they are the collector's items of the human race.

Such were the sorrows of wife Margaret vergh Gryffith, who, in the year 1588, in the month of May, in the town of Llangadfan, in Montgomeryshire, in the country of Wales, awoke one morning, stretched, rubbed her eyes to clear them of sleep, and felt (qual orrore!) a growth upon her forehead. At first a scaly eminence, a small rising at the very center of her brow; soon a horrid excrescence that no amount of dedicated picking, scraping, or nailed excavation could dislodge, so firm were its rootings. Daily it grew longer and larger in its girth, as though all of the young matron's energies were concentrated and refined to this one wicked purpose. Through salve and unguent she passed, through poultice and plaster, through the cook of cautery and the sizzle of scarification to the endless agitation of *concealment*. But there was no way to do it, no cap or snood, net or kerchief, hood or cowl to hide this . . . *horn*. Yes, at last it must be said. Margaret vergh Gryffith had grown a horn which stood priapically from her brow for a height of three inches, then curved downward toward her nose to crook just above her right eye—there, where there is nothing for it but to *see* it or shut forever her eyes and sit blind beneath her antler.

Imagine poor Margaret's shame, her altered sense of herself. See her devising more and more desperate articles and habits of concealment. It was of no use. As well hang a smoking brazier on the thing and walk abroad. The horn could not be hid! Wheresoever she faced, in whatever stance, however deep her crouch, it was the horn stood high and hard before her, rejecting all drapery, a lewd probe that announced to her Puritan contemporaries as the very cornified concretion of adultery, an adultery she did not commit.

Then were fiery sermons delivered in all the cathedrals of Wales, to which the people came, and listened, and trembled in their pews. As far away as London was Margaret vergh Gryffith "made readie to be seene" and led out upon platforms whilst men thundered and pointed; and alone in their boudoirs, women raised cold fearful fingertips to their foreheads, and shuddered.

Shame on you, London. Where was your bold surgeon in 1588 who would dare thrust to the fore of the lickerish crowd, to lead the horned woman away to his surgery, to amputate the hideous prong of packed and layered keratin from her head?

Ah, he jests at scars who never felt a wound.

How proud and easy we slide in our skin. Extensible, it stretches to fit our farthest reach, contracts to our least flicker, and all in silky silence. How our skin becomes us! Lucky is Man to have his hide.

Moreover, it is not the brain nor the heart that is the organ of recollection. It is the skin! For to gaze upon the skin is to bring to life the past.

Here, in the crook of this arm, where the loose skin lies in transverse folds, in this very place, she rested the back of her head, her hair so black and glossy I could see myself in the mass of it.

And from this lower lip she drew two drops of my blood, that I was glad to give her.

And look, this scar upon my cheek that marked the end of love between two brothers.

It is all here engraved, that which I was, that which I did, all the old stories, but now purified somehow, the commonplace washed away, rinsed of all that is ordinary, and glowing as they never did, even when they happened.

THE BELLY

Consider the aweto—embodiment of dietary indiscretion—which caterpillarlike creature burrows beneath the earth of New Zealand in search of a certain seed for which it lusts unceasingly. So unbounded is the aweto's craving for this seed that the aweto spurns all other nourishment, preferring starvation to any palatine concession. Ah, but no sooner has the hideous seed been found and ingested, than it germinates—sprouting, branching, growing with such zest as to quickly exceed the capability of the aweto to expel it in either direction. Soon the malevolent fungus can be seen emerging from the mouth of the aweto, elongating, dividing, thrusting spurs through the aweto's brain. Now the aweto has the look of an anguished elk. It is thus, crammed and bursting, that the aweto dies, its corpse a mere fingerling upon the burgeoning meal-beast.

Let us properly go from the instruction of the aweto to the stomach in its abdominal residence. Let us go with fit trepidation, with all due ceremony, for we are entering upon imperial ground.

Here then is the abdomen, a vessel where secrets hatch, chemistries, dark rituals. Scan, please, from the twin sails of the diaphragm that catch the winds from the north, to the sturdy dinghy of the pelvis rocking atop the thighs. No shield protects the abdomen, no scale or plated deck. It is only soft flesh, the touchiest of parts—and studded with the sad small stump of the navel, pathetic twist, all that is left of the primal separation, knotted lest our animus leak from us with an obscene little noise.

Within row the organs, slaves in a galley. The stomach, that succulent flared bag hung from the esophagus that drapes across the upper abdomen, tailing out into the intestine, is the brute who wields the lash. On its either side are the massive bulwarks of the liver and the spleen. They have not the stomach's slither, its grind, but, fortresses, they stand guard, thunderous and glowering in their opposite diaphragmatic recesses. Sliding between, the ravenous stomach holds upward its open mouth. It is the least refined of organs, a fetid, rank, and gaseous trough that knows but the pressure of fullness, the cavernous echo of emptiness—a pink, moist, hairless creature whose call is a belch and who responds to its ingests with delirious contractions and metallic bleeping. It is, all in all, an uncouth performance. Devoid of dream and imagination, lacking the lambent finesse of the heart, ignorant of the sweet language of the sex organs, the stomach sweats and steams and grunts most happily.

But let no man snub his stomach. Come, be very very kind to the stomach. You had better.

In repose, the stomach is a J-shaped flaccid sack, and it thus follows that there is a greater and a lesser curvature. Above is the cardia, below the pylorus. In the middle is the capacious antrum through which food traverses an imaginary channel, the *Magenstrasse*. Two layers of muscle, one longitudinal, the other circular, envelop the stomach. These muscle layers, aroused by the presence of food in the antrum, are thrown into vigorous contortion. Waves of peristalsis erupt in the cardia and ripple downward to spend themselves at the pylorus. Ridges are raised, indentations cut, as this fierce energy is transmitted from cell to cell, advancing upon the tissues in a broad front, engulfing them. The whole corpus of the stomach contracts, squeezing, battering, bruising its contents in an orgy of trituration. No stung horse shudders and rears so mightily.

Deeper lies the mucosa—to the naked eye, a pleated velvety sheet that undulates upon the muscles. Seen beneath the microscope, the mucosa is a vast sea of identical cells from each of which there drip the hydrochloric acid and enzymes that sterilize, break down, and otherwise process what has been eaten. Here and there the cellular monotony is broken by the presence of a goblet cell, wherefrom oozes the mucus with which the stomach lining is coated lest the stomach lining be digested by its own secretion.

In many animals, birds most notably, the stomach has two compartments, the smaller of which is the crop. Given the absence of teeth, the bird swallows its dentition in the form of pebbles. These pebbles are held in the crop for the purpose of grinding the food before it is passed on as pulp to the main secretory chamber. It is said that in 1642 the English physiologist William Harvey, having observed hawks regurgitating the impacted rejectimenta of fur and bone, held his ear to the breast of an eagle and first heard the distant clinking of these little rocks. Intrepid Harvey to dare such an ogling of eagles, a hearkening to hawks.

The flow of gastric juice—a now and then affair—is stimulated by the sight, taste, and smell of food, and as well by rage, especially the suppressed kind, and by all variety of private *Sturm und Drang*. The messages arrive at the stomach aboard the vagus nerves. These are two large trunks that wander from the base of the brain, emerge through holes at the bottom of the skull, and course

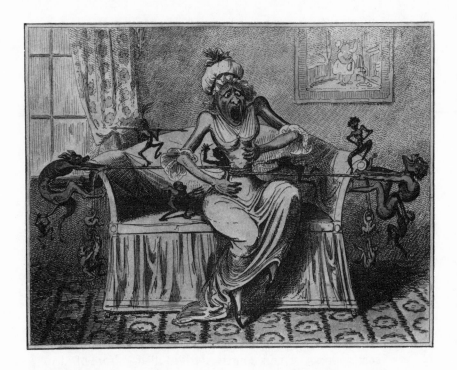

through the neck and thorax before spraying out upon the
stomach in a wild extravaganza. To these signals the great
fermenting vat responds, opening or closing the faucets of
secretion, enhancing or stilling the force of peristalsis, con-
trolling the sphincters at the stomach's inlet and outlet.

Thus does foraging man eat of the dawn-colored peach.
Thus does he digest, absorb, assimilate, and make the rosy
peach his own, divesting himself of the residue as excre-
ment. There is poetry in such an anatomy, such a chemistry, and so it does not astonish that an organ so tirelessly
dedicated to the care and sustenance of the entire body
should have appealed to physicians over the centuries as a
locus possessed of charmed healing properties.

Of greatest fame is the bezoar. In the stomach of certain

animals there happens the occasional formation of a stone, a concretion built from the ground-up products of ingestion upon which a shell of lime or salts of magnesium has been overlaid. Such bezoars have been found even in man. Composed of vegetable matter and hair, the fibers wed themselves into a Gordian knot. Once formed, the bezoar invites the layering of further encrustation, the whole being compressed into greater and greater solidity by the working of the stomach, until at last the growth has reached a size such as to prevent either its passage into the intestine or its retrograde ejection by vomiting. There the bezoar sits, like six green apples, rolling about monstrously, blocking up the *Magenstrasse* and otherwise interfering with the good order of things.

All homage to the ancient Persian doctors who recognized the curative and antidotal powers of these heavy *Lumpenfleischen* and made sweet use of them to forfend against shipwreck, to bring rain, and to escort women safely through the shoals of childbirth. As an antidote for poison, the bezoar was unexcelled, perhaps still is. Until recent political events contrived to rid their culture of ideologically heretical truths, the Chinese wore bezoars set into rings, which rings one sucked whenever he believed himself poisoned.

Watch a snake swallowing a rabbit whole, or a sea gull downing a bass intact, and you will know that man is not alone in his cavalier treatment of the stomach. The entire animal world is of the same reprehensible sangfroid. Nor is it any wonder that we offend the stomach in our language, as it is the stomach that accounts for the offenses to our person. *I shall no longer stomach your insults* makes clear our outrage, and heralds, too, the production to excess of hydrochloric acid. Prodded by tension, rage, angst, the floodgates open and a veritable torrent of corrosion flows from the stomach lining to slosh in scalding puddles across membranes, inflaming, burning, eroding—finally ulcerating.

It is as if one had swallowed nettles. Jaws are deep embedded. A sandpaper tongue licks lavishly at flesh. The stomach is devouring itself; it is become Samson, bent on avulsing the very pillars of the body—even if this must mean the stomach's own destruction.

Gone is the acid's healthy intermittency; a river is born, overwhelming the neutralizing effect of the alkaline saliva and the protective lubricant of mucus over which the gastric juice would slide harmlessly in happier times. Rubor, Tumor, Dolor, Calor (Redness, Swelling, Pain, Heat), the Four Horsemen of Peptic Apocalypse come riding hard, galloping across the midriff, pillaging, raping tissue, laying waste. On and on they stampede, unchecked by antacid, surcease, even sleep, their lust sated only by the triple calamities of Obstruction, Hemorrhage, and Perforation.

The crater enlarges. Tissue close by grows wooden and thick, blocking the outlet of the stomach with walls of scar. Now you vomit, and the excavation deepens. An artery is laid bare at the base. It too is eaten away and there is bleeding, often massive. Great gobbets of blood are tossed from the mouth, or slide in tarry rivers to be discharged from the bowel. You are pale and sweaty with shock. At last, the fifth column marches. One cell too many has been worn away, and the wall of the gut is penetrated! The acid bubbles forth to burn and soil the peritoneum. It is through such a punched-out hole that we plunge to escape the injustices of our lives, our lovelessness, business reverses, resentment of the mortal condition. Now pain graduates to agony. A stake has been hammered into the abdomen. One must remain perfectly still, for with the slightest movement more acid lips the ulcer's rim. More spillage. New splendors of pain. Breath itself is feared. A hiccough might topple the brain into madness. Untreated, the peritonitis rages and you are blessed by relief only in death.

Master of deception, the stomach is the archetype of the enemy within. Slung athwart the upper abdomen like a slowly fattening worm, straining upward in passive receipt, the stomach dwells, grinding its cud in blunt rumination. Is the world undone? A retarded serf, the stomach simply pursues its banality. Does the sun fall from the sky? The stomach cares not a fig. Quakes the earth? Ho hum. The stomach's contentment bears only upon its content, from moment to moment. Yet, interrupt for a time the care and feeding of this sack of appetite, do it insult with no matter how imagined a slight, then turns the worm to serpent that poisons the intellect for thought, the soul for poetry, the heart for love.

Most peptic ulcers are less than half an inch in diameter, about ten cents' worth really, and occur within two inches of the pylorus, most often in the first portion of the intestine, the duodenum, into which the raw gastric juice is poured, and which lacks the protective mucus the stomach is supplied. One out of every ten American men will earn a peptic ulcer at some time in his life. Most susceptible are bus drivers, taxi drivers, business executives, and foremen. But in the vast majority of cases, the ailment is rightly viewed as a mere annoyance, for these ulcers have a strong tendency to heal spontaneously no matter what the sufferer does, and given a regimen of antacids, bland diet, and an avoidance of stress and hunger, the ulcer fairly races closed, until all that is left is a small scar visible only as a tiny defect on the x-ray. Yet, while there has been a marked increase in the incidence of peptic ulcer in the past hundred years, there has been a steady decline in the occurrence of cancer of the stomach. It is as though the gentlemanly stomach, its honor ever inflamed, would accept a palpable hit rather than insist upon a mortal wound.

Living with your stomach is not unlike living with a petulant spouse upon whose bounty you must depend. Peevish, for example, even spiteful, is the abhorrence of the stomach for motion. Was there ever a man who did not yearn for the ocean voyage, who has not pictured himself, legs braced upon the slanting deck, cap set low and tight against the wind, who has not ached to feel the gleaming elements washing him with their detergent miracle? But let him, seduced by visions of traveling skies, sign on for such a dream, and then let him glide from view, and the wine of adventure sours to gall and wormwood by foulest alchemy. Who was to be rocked gently in the cradle of the deep is now pitched and rolled in the slather from the sea's numberless running mouths, and the god of nausea, insatiable Neptune, receives, unappeased, the gifts of the stomach.

Wherefore this distrust of movement? Is not man bounced from very egg, very spermhood, upon the gossamer membranes of tube and uterus? Is he not thereafter dandled and tumbled to rest his ease? Does man make love absolutely still? My God, does not the earth itself spin in the void? Ah, perverse stomach, so quick to take umbrage at the tilting of a mere spoonful's fluid in the deepest chambers of the ear. But hush. I must say no more. To speak against the stomach is to invite calamity, and even now I sense the first wamblings of bloffoblagia in my middle.

But, Capricious Stomach, listen. Why make of pregnancy a bilious wobble? For what should be, from that secret soft sublimest slippage of the moorings until the splashing of the anchor a three-quarter-year sojourn upon serenest seas, becomes an ungainly lurch from basin to pot, as you, Sulky Stomach, turn violet morn to greenest midnight. Despised alike are the sight of food and the horrid goat-footed Impregnator. Stomach, Stomach, wherefore this spite, this discompassion, this fury to discommode? Is it that, having enjoyed none of the ecstasies of conjugation, thou art now solicited to wet-nurse the product thereof? To eat for two?

Stomach, I must agree, thou art ill-used by love's appetite.

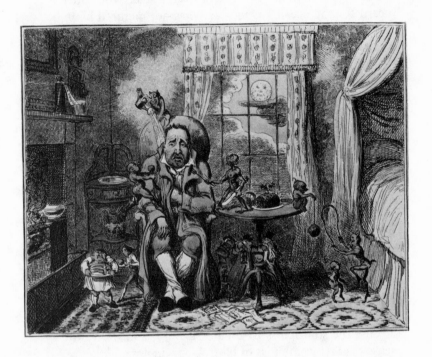

Little was known of the physiology of the stomach and its infamy—the peptic ulcer—until the nineteenth century. Among those few that guessed, one was Amatus Lusitanus, a famous Marrano physician of sixteenth-century Spain. In 1548, while browsing in a bookshop, Amatus met an old friend and fellow doctor, Azariah dei Rossi. Azariah was then being persecuted for refusing to renounce his Judaism, and the two men had experienced some estrangement because of the Inquisition. Still, after being greeted by Amatus, Azariah requested a stall-side consultation, for Azariah had not been feeling well at all. Azariah was then thirty-five years old and of ascetic build—a true leptosome. In the refuge of the bookshop, the differences between the two doctors dissolved, doubtless the accumulation of printed wisdom about them aiding in this reconciliation.

Azariah, responding to Amatus' questions: yes, he experienced pain in his upper abdomen; yes, it was worse at night; yes, the pain was accompanied by growling noises from deep within his belly; yes, he was often seized by *fames canina*, hunger of a dog.

Too early by three hundred years to suspect that his friend had grown a duodenal ulcer, but acting from the deep well of intuition that is said to be the property of the gifted physician, Amatus laid blame upon the tensions under which Azariah was forced to live in Inquisitorial Spain. This, reasoned Amatus, plus an intense preoccupation with study, had conspired to disrupt Azariah's equilibrium and to bring him to his present state of ruin. Amatus prescribed a diet of cooked fruit and vegetables, white bread with caraway seeds (to defend against flatulence), and the soup of chicken. Beans and other legumes, as well as fried foods, were to be avoided, and wine allowed only if diluted with cold barley water. There was to be sufficient sleep, little study, and only so much sex as necessary to refresh oneself. And, of course, Azariah was to apply to his body an unguent of goose fat, vinegar, and oil of roses.

Four months later Azariah reported to Amatus a complete recovery, and thereafter Azariah lived and worked in excellent health for thirty years.

My grandmother, who never went to medical school, could have diagnosed and prescribed as well. In particular, I point to the use of chicken soup. As in all discoveries, timing is essential. Thus it is Amatus who is honored in the gilded manuscripts of medicine, whereas Becky Schneider is remembered not even by most of her kin. It is ever thus. But I would deny no praise to Amatus, who, as long ago as the sixteenth century, divined that the pain in Spain came mainly from the strain.

In 1824, the English scientist William Prout discovered that the stomach produced hydrochloric acid. Prior to

Prout, almost nothing of the mechanism of digestion was known. The stomach was thought of as a kind of mill, a fermenting wine vat, a stew pan. A Renaissance text announces that into the stomach are let down the aliments as alkalescent flesh, rancescent fat, and acescent vegetables. Here they are digested in a heat equal to that of the liver, macerated and corrupted into a liquid putrescence. All respect to the scholars of the Enlightenment, but there is nothing more depressant to the appetite than a reading of the early manuscripts on the subject of digestion, among which *De Vomitu et Nausea* and *De Monstris* are the most disgusting examples.

Science has often been served at the expense of the hapless. Progress is more the ancient dance of the hunter and the hunted than the guileless strivings of God-fearing man. So it has been with gastroenterology, whose brazenest idol is one William Beaumont.

In the year 1822, in the Michigan Territories, fur was king. John Jacob Astor had conceived his scheme of harvesting the mammals of North America with whose polished hair he intended to bedeck all of Europe. To this purpose, he had dispatched squadrons of militia, by land and water, to set up trading posts throughout the area. Trappers were enlisted from among the settlers. Alexis St. Martin, eighteen years old and adventurous, was one such husky fellow. William Beaumont was a young Army doctor assigned to the military post in the trading center of Fort Mackinac.

On June 6 of that year, as St. Martin stood by his pile of scooped-out muskrats in the company store, a musket was accidentally discharged no more than a yard away. The shot struck the boy in his left side, blowing open a hole in his stomach—a hole that was never to close, but which, like a stigma of martyrdom, would remain unhealed forever. A steady rivulet of gastric juice welled from the rim of his hole, and at its base could be seen the spongy hillocks of the very lining of the stomach itself. It was a shot to be heard around the scientific world.

William Beaumont was summoned to tend the wound. He knelt beside the pile of skins upon which the boy lay, and gazed long and deep into the bloody mangle, seeing reflected in that crimson swim his power and his glory. Not Salome nor Lady Macbeth more eagerly imbrued her trembling hands with gore. Beaumont trimmed and patched and stitched with all his considerable art, for he was a good, an honorable, surgeon. And it came to pass that the boy St. Martin recovered. The torn flesh healed, almost, it shrank, threw itself up into hard lips of scar about the permanent shriek of the wound, the new mouth that was to become for St. Martin a trap as toothed as any he had set in the many-beavered forest. For two years, each day, Beaumont tied pieces of meat, potatoes, bread, fruit, and vegetables to a silk string, and these he lowered into the wound, pressing them deep within the entrails of his "patent digester." He would withdraw these tasties at varying intervals, to record in his notebook the exact state of the particle's decomposition.

Imagine poor St. Martin, cowering in a corner, pleading with the demonic doctor, the man who had *saved his life*— at first silently, not wishing to offend his benefactor (now his master), then openly whimpering: "Oh, not the string. Not the string. Not again, please."

For almost three years Beaumont kept St. Martin in thrall, playing upon the boy's natural gratitude—until, fingered, instilled, strung beyond endurance, St. Martin ran away. The ingrate defected.

A terrier after his rat, Beaumont hounded his St. Martin from village to village, yipping at his heels, the Skulker Obsessed. Flask and pipette in one hand, dreadful notebook in the other, Beaumont at last found and recaptured St. Martin, "worthless, nekkid, and drunk," and wrenched him from his land and family for another five-year tour of duty. Envision poor St. Martin, in tavern with glass at lip, or tending his traps in the forest primeval, or abed with his Indian squaw. He glances up, distracted by a movement at the periphery of his vision, and sees there the hated, eager, assiduous Beaumont, one hand extended to catch the drops of gastric juice welling from the notorious wound.

Shame on you, Dr. Beaumont. And all praise to you, too.

Then think upon the aweto, ye carefree, rash, imprudent men. In the ribbed darkness of the body, Belly dwells a prisoner, fed or starved as suits his jailer, at whose whim he is bludgeoned by leaden dumplings, or is with harshest horseradish seared. At once a captive, yet warder too, Belly holds within his hollow squirm the very keys that would unlock him to rampage most awful. Then he turns upon his keeper; a fever heats the prison; it may burn to the ground. Belly knows he dies with the rest. Yet he is beyond caring. No common jailbird, this Belly, but . . . God in chains!— nudging, goading, according to his grand design. Take care to worship—lest He eat you, and your children, and your children's children, and put an end to the race of man.

THE CORPSE

[Homage to Sir Thomas Browne]

Shall I tell you once more how it happens? Even though you know, don't you?

You were born with the horror stamped upon you, like a fingerprint. All these years you have lived you have known. I but remind your memory, confirm the fear that has always been prime. Yet the facts have a force of their insolent own.

Wine is best made in a cellar, on a stone floor. Crush grapes in a barrel such that each grape is burst. When the barrel is three-quarters full, cover it with a fine-mesh cloth, and wait. In three days, an ear placed low over the mash will detect a faint crackling, which murmur, in two more days, rises to a continuous giggle. Only the rendering of fat or a forest fire far away makes such a sound. It is the song of fermentation! Remove the cloth and examine closely. The eye is startled by a bubble on the surface. Was it there and had it gone unnoticed? Or is it newly come?

But soon enough more beads gather in little colonies, winking and lining up at the brim. Stagnant fluid forms. It begins to turn. Slow currents carry bits of stem and grape meat on voyages of an inch or so. The pace quickens. The level rises. On the sixth day, the barrel is almost full. The teem must be poked down with a stick. The air of the cellar is dizzy with fruit flies and droplets of smell. On the seventh day, the fluid is racked into the second barrel for aging. It is wine.

Thus is the fruit of the earth taken, its flesh torn. Thus is it given over to standing, toward rot. It is the principle of corruption, the death of what is, the birth of what is to be.

You are wine.

SHE: Is he dead, then?

HE: I am sorry.

SHE: Oh, God.

HE: I should like to ask . . . because of the circumstances of your husband's death, it would be very helpful . . . to do . . . an autopsy.

SHE: Autopsy? No, no, not that. I don't want him cut up.

Better to have agreed, madam. We use the trocar on all, autopsied or merely embalmed. You have not heard of the suction trocar? Permit me to introduce you to the instrument.

A hollow steel rod some two feet in length, one end, the tip, sharp, pointed; to the other end there attaches rubber tubing, which tubing leads to the sink; near this end the handle, sculpted, the better to grip with; just inside the tip, holes, a circle of them, each opening large enough to admit the little finger or to let a raisin pass. This is the trocar.

A man stands by the table upon which you lie. He opens the faucet in the sink, steps forward, raises the trocar. It is a ritual spear, a gleaming emblem. Two inches to the left and two inches above your navel is the place of entry. (Feel it on yourself.) The technician raises this thing and aims for the spot. He must be strong, and his cheeks shake with the thrust. He grunts.

Wound most horrible! It is a goring.

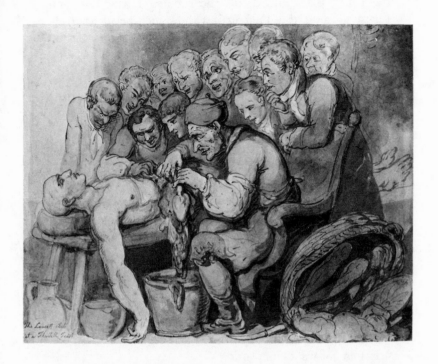

The head of the trocar disappears beneath the skin.
Deeper and deeper until the body wall is penetrated. Another thrust, and he turns the head north. First achieved is
the stomach, whose stringy contents, food just eaten, are
sucked into the holes. A three-inch glass connector interrupts the rubber tubing. Here one is spectator as the yield
rushes by. Can you identify particular foods? Beets are
easy, and licorice. The rest is merely . . . gray.

Look how the poker rides—high and swift and lubri-
cious. Several passes, and then the trocar is drawn expertly
back until the snout is barely hidden beneath the skin. The
man takes aim again, this time for the point of the chin, he
says. Then he dives through the mass of the liver, across
the leaf of the diaphragm, and into the right chambers of

the heart. Black blood fills the tubing. Thrust and pull, thrust and pull, thunking against the spine, the staves of the ribs, shivering the timbers, the brute bucking as it rides the magnificent forearm of the Licensed Embalmer in high rodeo.

The heart is empty. The technician turns the tool downward, into the abdomen once more. Now are the intestines pierced, coil upon coil, collapsing their gas and their juice to the sink. It is brown in the glass connector. Thunk, thunk, the rod smites the pelvis from within. The dark and muffled work is done: the scrotum is skewered, the testicles mashed, ablaze with their billion whiptail jots. All, all into the sink—and then to the sewer. This is the ultimate suck.

The technician disconnects the tubing from the sink, joins the tubing to a pump. He fires the motor; preservative fluid boils up, streams into the trocar, thence to thorax and abdomen.

The trocar is doubly clever.

HE: Urea combines with the phenol to make plastic. We, in effect, plasticize the body.
SHE: I do not want him plastic.
HE: It's only a word.
SHE: Jesus, words.
HE: There is the problem of the mouth.
SHE: Jesus, problems.
HE: It is all words, all problems. Trust me; I see. I . . . am . . . a physician. I really know, don't you see?
SHE: All right, then. The mouth. Tell me.

Our technician forces the mouth shut, holds it there, assessing. Buckteeth are a problem, he says. Sometimes you have to yank them to get the mouth closed. He removes his hand, and the mandible drops again. Now he takes a large flat needle. It is S-shaped, for ease of grasping. A length of white string hangs through the eye of this needle. He

132

draws back the bottom lip with thumb and forefinger. He passes the needle into the lower gum. Needle and string are pulled through and out, and the lip allowed to rest. Next, the upper lip is held away, and the needle is passed up into the groove at the crest of the upper gum, thence to the left nostril, through the nasal septum into the right nostril, finally plunging back into that groove and once again to the mouth. This stitchery will not be seen. Pledgets of cotton are inserted to fill out a sag here, a droop there, lest the absence of teeth or turgor be noticed.

What? No penny enslotted here for Charon? No bite of honey cake for mad Cerberus?

No. Only cotton.

About this invented fullness the jaws are drawn to as the string is tied. One square knot is followed by two grannies. Prevents slippage, Death's tailor says. Gone is all toothy defiance. In its place, there is only the stuffed pout of anything filled too much. Now the plastic caps are inserted beneath the eyelids—pop, pop. And here—hold still—we are ready for cosmetics.

The case is opened importantly. It is of alligator hide, imitation of this. Within are shelves for the jars, slots for the brushes, as many as the vanity Death's whore requires. The technician selects three jars. Red, yellow, blue: daubs a bit of each on the palette; mixes, turns, and wipes—until the color of your skin is matched. More blue for Negroes, says he; less yellow and more blue for them. He has said something unarguable—and is now quiet. Many a sidelong glance later, he is ready. He steps to the head of the table and applies the paint, massages the color into the skin of face and hands. This is what shows, he says. And one must do, but not overdo, he says. At last our fellow approves. How lovely the morning, pockless glow! It is a wholesome look—a touch of evening blue in the hollows of the lids. Oh, yes, art is truly bottled sunshine.

Who, but a moment ago, was huffing rider of the belly is

133

now artist, configuring Death, shaping it. He has rebuilt a ravaged chin, replaced an absent nose, he says. Give him enough plaster and a bit of paint and he can make a man, he says. I wait for him to lean over and blow into these nostrils. He can make anything except life, he says.

Thus combed and shaved (lemon-scented Colgate is nice) and powdered, the corpse gleams, a marquis upon ruched velvet, banked with fierce forced blossoms.

SHE: Embalming belittles death.
HE: On the contrary, art dignifies. It is the last passion. For both fellows, don't you know?
SHE: But there must be some other way. As for myself, mind you, I prefer to be of use. I have made arrangements that my body be given to a medical school for dissection. I carry this little card that so states. In case of accident.
HE: A gesture in the grand style. You join a gallant band. So many are concerned with the appearance of the flesh, leaving ill-considered its significance. Well . . . its usefulness.

Forty feet long, four wide, and seven deep is THE TANK. It is set into the ground at the very bottom of the medical school. If Anatomy be the firstborn of Medicine, then the tank is its sunken womb. Here at the very center of stench it lies; here is the bite of embalming fluid sharpest. Tears overwhelm the eyes. The tank demands weeping of this kind. It is lidded, covered by domed metal, handle at apex, like a casserole of chow mein.

Let me remove this lid. Behold! How beautiful they are, the bodies. With what grace and pomp each waits his turn. Above the fluid, a center rod, like a closet rod, suspends them in a perfect row; forty soldiers standing in the bath, snug as pharaohs, only heads showing, all facing, obediently, the same way.

Come, walk the length of the tank. We review these warriors who, by their bearing, salute us. Arteries have been pumped full of fluid. It helps the flesh to sink, lest feet float to the top in embarrassing disarray. Thus weighted, the bodies swim readily to erect posture. Upon each head, worn with a certain nonchalance, are the tongs, the head-dress of this terrible tribe. The hooks of the tongs are inserted one into each ear, then sunk home by pulling on the handle. Each set of tongs is then hung from the center rod by a pulley. In this way the bodies can be skimmed back and forth during the process of selection or to make room for another.

We end skin overcoats on a rack.

A slow current catches the brine and your body sways ever so slightly, keeping time. This movement stirs the slick about your shoulders. Iridescent colors appear, and little chunks of melt, shaken off in annoyance, it seems, bob up and down.

Does some flame far below, at the center of the earth, thus bring this tank to lazy boil? Or is it the heat from hell? Look. A dead fly floats, one wing raised in permanent effort at extrication. A fly? Well, of course. There is food here.

It is wine.

SHE: I want nothing done. Let him be put in the ground as he is.

HE: You are distraught. Perspective. What you need is perspective. Listen. Outside the rain is falling, soft as hair. [A pause] No toilette, then?

Dead, the body is somehow more solid, more massive. The shrink of dying is past. It is as though only moments before a wind had kept it aloft, and now, settled, it is only what it is—a mass, declaring itself, an ugly emphasis. Almost at once the skin changes color, from pink-highlighted yellow to gray-tinted blue. The eyes are open and lackluster; something, a bright dust, had been blown away, leaving the globes smoky. And there is an absolute limpness. Hours later, the neck and limbs are drawn up into a semiflexion, in the attitude of one who has just received a blow to the solar plexus.

One has.

Even the skin is in rigor, is covered with goose bumps. Semen is forced from the penis by the contraction of muscle. The sphincters relax, and the air is poisonous with loosed sewage. Colder and colder grows the flesh, as the last bit of warmth disperses. Now you are meat, meat at room temperature.

Examine once more the eyes. How dull the cornea, this globe bereft of tension. Notice how the eyeball pits at the pressure of my fingernail. Whereas the front of your body is now drained of color, the back, upon which you rest, is found to be deeply violet. Even here, even now, gravity works upon the blood. In twenty-four hours, your untended body resumes its flaccidity, resigned to this everlasting posture.

You stay thus.

You do not die all at once. Some tissues live on for minutes, even hours, giving still their little cellular shrieks, molecular echoes of the agony of the whole corpus. Here and there a spray of nerves dances on. True, the heart stops; the blood no longer courses; the electricity of the brain sputters, then shuts down. Death is now *pronounceable*. But there are outposts where clusters of cells yet shine, besieged, little lights blinking in the advancing darkness. Doomed soldiers, they battle on. Until Death has secured the premises all to itself.

The silence, the darkness, is not for long. That which was for a moment dead leaps most sumptuously to life. There is a busyness gathering. It grows fierce.

There is to be a feast. The rich table has been set. The board groans. The guests have already arrived, numberless bacteria that had, in life, dwelt in saprophytic harmony with their host. Their turn now! Charged, they press against the membrane barriers, break through the new softness, sweep across plains of tissue, devouring, belching gas —a gas that puffs eyelids, cheeks, abdomen into bladders of murderous vapor. The slimmest man takes on the bloat of corpulence. Your swollen belly bursts with a ripping sound, followed by a long mean hiss.

And they are at large! Blisters appear upon the skin, enlarge, coalesce, blast, leaving brownish puddles in the declivities. You are becoming gravy. Arriving for the banquet late, of course, and all the more ravenous for it, are the twin sisters Calliphora and raucous Lucilia, the omnipresent greenbottle flies, their costumes metallic sequins. Their thousands of eggs are laid upon the meat, and soon the mass is wavy with the humped creamy backs of maggots nosing, crowding, hungrily absorbed. Gray sprays of fungus sprout in the resulting marinade, and there lacks only a mushroom growing from the nose.

At last—at last the bones appear, clean and white and dry. Reek and mangle abate; diminuendo the buzz and crawl. All, all is eaten. All is done. Hard endlessness is here even as the revelers abandon the skeleton.

You are alone, yet again.

HE: Come, come, we are running out of time. How, at last, would you dispose of your husband? You must make a decision.

SHE: Why must I?

HE: Because you are the owner of the body. It is your possession.

SHE: Oh, cremation, dammit. I'm sick of this business.

HE: Brava! Man is pompous in the grave, splendid in ashes.

SHE: A smaller package to mail.

HE: You are doing the right thing, I assure you. The physiognomy does not endure in the grave. There is no identity. Cremation is tidy. I can see that you abhor the slough of putrefaction. Who wouldn't?

To the prettiness again. . . .

The good fellow slides you into the oven, and ignites the fire. If you are burned in your casket, an exhaust fan sucks away the wood ash, until there is only your body. He observes through a peephole at the back of the oven. Now he turns off the exhaust, and lets the flames attack the body. Three hours later, at two thousand degrees Fahrenheit, it is done. The oven is turned off, is let cool overnight. The next day a rear door is opened, and the ashes are examined. Intact pieces of bone are pulverized with a mallet. With a little broom the residue is whisked into an urn. The operator is fastidious, down to smallest bits of dust.

The modern urn is no garnished ossuary, but a tin can indistinguishable from that which holds coffee by the pound. It is unadorned. Pry open the lid and see the expensive white doily, of the best embossed paper, creased like a priest's napkin. Unfold it, and gaze upon the contents. Shocking! They are not ashes but chunks of bone, and recognizable as such. Some as big as your thumbnail, chalky, charred. A tin of cinders. Coals and calx—with the odor of smoke and the semen-smell of cooked bone.

SHE: How do I know that it is my husband's ashes that you give me? That they are not his but some other's—an old woman's, a dog's?

HE: A vile and baseless suspicion. Now, in the matter of the cremains . . .

SHE: The what?

HE: Your husband's cremains.

SHE: His ashes?

HE: Yes. Many bereaved find it a soothing term, less harsh than . . . you know . . .

But you are right to question.

Who knows the fate of his bones? His ashes? To what purpose tamp them into sad sepulchral pitchers? I have seen the cremation of two, even three, together. Later, the ashes were shoveled into cans in equal amounts, and labeled. Why not? Great religions have flourished on more spurious assumptions. The idea is not new. Were not the ashes of Achilles mingled with those of his lover Patroclus? Ah, you say, it is one thing to burn lovers, then fondly stir their ashes together; quite another to have one's urn-fellows selected at random.

Yet are not all our greatest intimacies merest chance?

HE: Have you considered the disposition of the ashes?

SHE: The toilet?

HE: I am afraid, madam, that we have reached an impasse. You prefer neither cremation nor embalming. You are repelled alike by anatomical dissection and the moist relentment of putrefaction. Why don't you admit that you are ashamed of death? You think it is a disgrace to be dead.

SHE: That's it. Yes. A disgrace. That's it exactly.

HE: Exactly, yes.

SHE: If you know everything, then what is your choice? For yourself?

HE: That is not the point.

Ah, but it is the point. Listen. On the banks of the Hudson, midway between Manhattan and Montreal, squats the lizard town of Troy. In the back room of Moriarity's Saloon, the November meeting of the Druids of Eld is taking place. Harry Bascomb rises to deliver the invocation:

"From insomnia as from bad dreams, from lack of love, from waiting so long you forget why, from enlargement of the prostate, from running out of coal, from constipation, from a sniveling son and a daughter who flunks Deportment, from the pox and from the gout, from a grave full of worms—in Moriarity's, in the woes of day and the throes of night, O Lord, deliver us."

This is followed by the ineffably sad sound of men trying to laugh together.

"The subject for tonight is what to do with your mortal remains. You first, Georgie."

Georgie assumes a leprechaun stoop and a high Irish voice. "I want me heart cut out and placed in a little silver box," he says, "with napkins and red candle wax all around. The rest ye can cast on terra damnata, and piss on it."

"You're next, Doc. Surely you've learned from the dying whispers of your fellow men?"

"Nothing. Nothing."

"What? A physician? Sawbones? Nothing? We can endure your hideous facts."

The doctor shivers despite the warmth of the saloon, and hugs his chest with his arms. He is fresh from debate with next of kin, weary, weary. There is a stain on his vest more terrible than the Ancient Mariner's eye.

"I want," he begins, "to be buried—unembalmed and unboxed—at the foot of a tree. Soon I melt and seep into the ground, to be drawn up by the roots. Straight to the top, strung in the crown, answering the air. There would be the singing of birds, the applause of wings."

"Fed to a tree? All right, then. But a cow would do the tree more good."

Then all sing:

> *O what shall be done with our dead, old boys?*
> *We'll run out of ground very soon.*
> *Why, pack 'em in straw for a bed, old boys,*
> *And freight 'em straight off to the moon.*
>
> *O what shall we do with our dead, old boys?*
> *It seems a shame to waste 'em.*
> *So after your tears are shed, old boys,*
> *Why, spit 'em and roast 'em and taste 'em.*

Then all drink their wine.
Wine?

III
ESSAYS

BALD!

What plague is this that so thrives in the night a whole forest is notoriously laid waste? It is a smoldering of the dark hours—infection! The bedroom air steams with pestilence. By dawn the rigor has passed, the fever broken, and cold gray light is witness to a rumpled pillow bestrewn with the Fallen and the Shed.

It is Baldness that rages thus.

O Scalp, Scalp, wilt thou not bleed, not scream from this murderous depilation? Behold, thou art scythed and give no sign save a silence from nape to brow.

To the mirror. Oh, God. The comb trembles! A pass, tentative, light, from occiput forward. Now you hold the comb aloft at the window, through which indifferent morning bestows light in whose lidless glare you see the carnage of the night. Desperate lips tell the mournful numbers. Twenty-eight! Twenty-eight corpselets hanging limp between the teeth. And even as you watch, twenty-nine and thirty, made airborne by some tardy gust, rock sinkward.

O wild punching of the air! O damn and damn!

Frantic fingers forage among the survivors. You search for tomahawk wounds, fissures, all the lacerations and gougings of assault. There is nothing. All is smooth. All is still. Barren. A curse has come and passed, leaving no trace. Ah, lion unmaned, cock uncombed.

Your fingertips speculate back and forth upon the apex of your noggin. It has an obscene feel. One is joyless playing with himself *here*. You incline your head forward; your eye strains: an impossible angle. A pinkness flashes into view, and the horror is confirmed. Pink!

A punishment, you think. One has gazed too long on low delights.

Hair today, gone tomorrow, you say, and give a soldierly little smile. Yet you know that it is the joke and not the hair that is on you. Steady. You *will* look on the bright side. Good riddance, you say. Think of Absalom hanging by his hair from a tree. No such infringement for you. And what of Samson? Oh, God, *Samson*, you say weakly, and read in the pattern of those hairs in the sink the clarion message of power failing.

But, come, come, worrier, won't you think of all the time to be saved? At least half an hour a day of primping? And money? No haircuts, no combs, no brushes. No soap.

It is no use. You are shorn, forlorn. Delilahed. You lurch to the telephone to sound the alarm: Dermatologist! Barber! Quack shop! There is no rescue, no Column of Light Brigade. You grow old. You get ugly. And you get it all figured out: you lose your hair, you lose your *mind*.

What is it, this snatching that pains worse than gout, hurts worse than hernia? It is called by doctors alopecia—fox mange, that is, for it comes to elderly foxes even as it does to us. Nor is it news. In ancient Egypt Amenophis II, Rameses II, and even Nefertiti had it. Aristotle was bald, as was Julius Caesar. Let us learn:

Embedded in the deepest layer of the skin, the dermis, are nests of specialized cells: hair follicles. Here the bubbling of cell division is most intense, new cells forming along the periphery, crowding the older ones toward the center of the follicle. These flatten, attenuate, and turn into filaments of protein called *keratin*. It is this keratin, both the secretion of the follicle and that which it will become, that is the hair.

Lucky follicle. To have its destiny in its secretion. It is what the poet wants but seldom gets.

Longer and longer grows the hair. On and on spins the follicle gnome, its growth intermittent; for there are rest periods: the gnome nods, and the hair remains in these respites the same length.

The scalp of the young adult boasts between 100,000 and 150,000 of these strands. Ninety percent grow while ten percent rest. At a hectic four tenths of a millimeter per day, the hair grows, accumulating unto itself its daily measure of keratin. Beard hair, if left intact, can reach a length of some thirty centimeters, that of the scalp, much longer. Just how long is still a matter of dispute among trichologists. George Catlin, artist, went West to draw Indians, and reported back to a breathless world that it was not uncommon among the Crow tribe for a warrior's hair to fall five feet, brushing his heels as he walked. Long Hair, chief of the Crows, possessed the bravest follicles of all. His unbound tresses not only reached the ground but trailed after him for several feet. Less heroic but more accessible to view were the seven legendary Sutherland Sisters, displayed from town to town by patent medicine men. The unslung manes of these ladies cascaded to the insteps of their high-button shoes.

Long hair has always been construed as prima facie evidence for virility and power, while the bare scalp is a mark of degradation. Thus was the topknot taken in battle as a trophy of war—for he who possesses the hair of his slain enemy takes unto himself all the strength and courage of that foe. Not by Indians alone was such bushwhacking done, but by Scythians, Visigoths, and, yes, Maccabees as well. And prisoners, novice soldiers, traitors, and adulteresses alike were shaved to announce their ignominy. Along came Christianity to change shame into humility by having its monks plow their manes into tonsures. Still, there is nothing to indicate that it made a single baldy feel one whit better.

Will you not be comforted by the knowledge that, balding, you lose not the possibility of hair? Will it help to learn that the follicles, for some reason as yet unknown, involute, close down only? That they bank the fires of their mitosis, but do not perish? On rare occasions they may be roused from their long sleep to thrive once more. One must cultivate such tiny hopes. They are all you have.

Numberless are the unguents and poultices, the stoups and butters with which desperate man has rubbed his pate. Eau de Portugal, d'Égypte, de Chine—all in vain. To no avail electricity, vibration, massage, frightening, and the wearing of all manner of strange devices including hog's bladder, which folk wisdom was whispered to me by an indebted witch whose instructions were to wear for seven days and seven nights a fresh porcine urinary bladder as a yarmulke or capulet.

Actually, the entire body is covered with hair, save for the palms and soles, most of it being of the vellus type, that fine fuzz that can be seen in a good light. These are like the hairs that we wore in our embryonic life. It is only here and there that creatures affect a more conspicuous display, for purposes of either sexual attraction or specific protection. The bristles of the warthog are, after all, a distant-early-warning system, an exteriorized hypersense that instructs of friend, foe, or food nearby. And the tail-tuft of cattle? Despite the biological cynicism that insists that the tuft was developed as a kind of evolutional fly whisk, anyone knows what a coy cow can do to a bull with a flick—now here, now there.

Why not revise your thinking, adopt a Grecian Urn mentality? Seen hair is nice, but that unseen is nicer still.

Nothing is known about the cause of baldness. At a

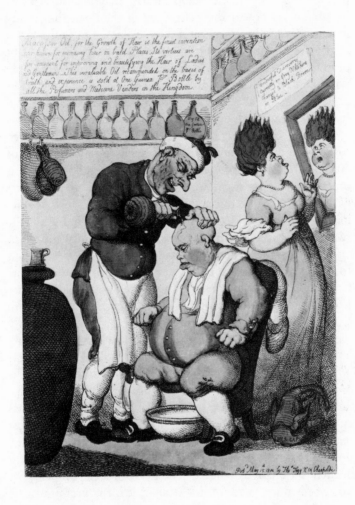

seventeenth-century symposium called *De Capelli e Peli*, on the scalp and hair, air pollution (miasmi pestiferi) was blamed for it. That hair follicles transplanted from another part of the body to the scalp flourish would indicate that hair-fall owes not to any deficiency of the tissue, nor is any impairment of the circulation thus suspected of fault. What *is* known is that androgen, the male sex hormone, must be present for baldness to develop, thus reinforcing the folk wisdom that baldness and virility go hand in hand. The replacement or addition of androgen by ingestion, injection, or smearing does nothing to delay or reverse the rate of balding. Only castration is effective. Thus did bald Aristotle gaze in envy at the flowing locks of the eunuchs of Athens. Nor is it known why, even as scalp hair is lost, otherwise hairless areas wax jungly. Witness the winglets of hair that sprout upon the shoulders of old men. Genes matter. As failed your father's, so fail yours. It is upon the reef of heredity that the fragile barque of beauty founders.

Why then this grieving over plait and lock? Does it comfort to learn baldness is the natural fate of the he-man? Come. With heart defiant, advance your naked pate proudly to the public eye. Hair is but a keepsake with sentimental value. We mourn its loss as we would any memento that must be surrendered to the earth. Therefore let your balditude be boldly proclaimed. Bald is beautiful!

There is comfort for man in the comradeship of the orangutan, the chimpanzee, the ouakari, and the stumptailed macaque, for they share in this unthatching. Nor has any of these beasts ever been observed to utter the least oath of shame or sorrow at such a falling out. Is not the dolphin bald? The whale? The dugong? What is clearly needed is a change of heart. The heart of a dugong is what you needs must have. In lieu of hair, it is the brain must be washed.

All right then, try philosophy. Be persuaded that it is in our nudity lies our greatness. In our nakedness are we most admirable. Who needs feathers? Of what use plumage when a blush will do? Still unconsoled? Well, then, obtain by any means practical, the bladder of a hog . . .

SMOKING

What some people will not do to assure themselves that they exist! A woman dabs her neck with perfume, then walks abroad. In the sensible cloud of droplets about her, she has created an extension of her corporeal self, and of her personality, too. With each inhalation, that which she may have but vaguely suspected, her *being*, is most indisputably confirmed. I am here, she sniffs happily. I am really here.

And whistlers. Even the air-hungriest asthmatic who has not the least idea where to place his pitch or tone, who plays blindman's buff with melodies no more intricate than *Mary Had a Little Lamb*, even such a one as this will walk the earth, lips pursed to a fine aperture, an expression of distraction upon his face as though he had just seen a vision. All the while from his feeble reed there issues a toneless beeping, a sorry complaint. It does not matter that the music he makes will not enter the living repertoire. No special color identifies it as baroque, flamenco, or twelve-tone; it is all of these and none of these. All about his head the whistler draws his helmet of sound. It is a private affair. Blowing out, he directs his notes within. The whistler himself but half attends the noise he makes. It is enough. He listens, and knows beyond all evidence to the contrary that he is there. His presence cannot be denied.

Thus do tenors and tuba players alike take the deep breath, set the vocal cords just so, and blast forth the good news of their existence. So, too, the child who climbs to the top of the slide, sits down, and makes ready to plummet. At the last moment he pauses, calls out to his mother. "Watch me!" he cries. And in her face he reads the success of his advertisement: *Here I am.*

I myself do it by smoking. And let no meddlesome man caution me against the extravagance, the injuriousness, of tobacco. I am addicted in a way more fundamental than any mere physiological craving. To deny me my smoke is to extinguish me as utterly as would death itself. It is to butt me into cold ashes.

Consider the act of smoking. It is constituted, is it not, of inhalation and exhalation? To draw deeply upon a cigarette, to fill the tracheobronchial tree with smoke, is to feed an empty space deep within, a space that twenty times a day cries out for appeasement. As nature abhors a vacuum, so does that cavern yearn for repletion. Should it, by some unhappy circumstance (you have run out of cigarettes in the dead of night), remain empty for too long a time, then the yearning becomes palpable. There is discomfort. The hollowness becomes an ache. One may perish of it.

I am not so vain, nor so uniquely neurotic, as to believe that I am alone in the world with such a hungry hole, a pit in search of something to enclose. Nor will mere fresh air suffice. For this interior sack is no mere biology, but an urbane bag for whom taste has been deliciously refined. It needs smoke. And smoke it shall have. Smoke is, after all, little enough. Time was when a man could, with the forthrightness of a child, enjoy a healthy expectoration, the passage of some audible flatus, or the scratching of his personals. But civilization has come to mean the narrowing down of what we are permitted to do in public. Little Bo-

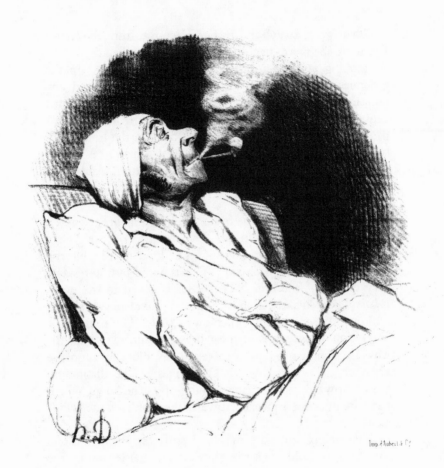

Peep has gone away, and in her place the Iron Maiden of Etiquette shepherds us toward good deportment.

Smoking is good for the dumpish heart; lights up the gloomies, don't you know? Let the innumerable sad circumstances of humiliations past, of stumbles yet to come, crowd in upon me; then, out of the night that covers me, I grope for that *thing* with which to tampon the leak in my soul. All at once there is the scratch of a match. A pretty flame breaks. It swings to the touch. Ignition! And there blows a very wind from paradise.

There are circuits in the brain and lung that are triggered by the shifting of gases in the blood. So goes our soughing: at the end of exhalation there is a small but measurable rise in the level of carbon dioxide. This is noted by the respiratory center of the brain. The order is issued to the lung: *inhale*. Oxygen is taken in, the carbon dioxide level falls. In a moment it will rise again. Now: *exhale*. The muscles of expiration, those strips of meat between and overlying the ribs, are commanded to contract. They close in upon the chest cage, compressing it. The leaves of the diaphragm billow upward, further encroaching upon the lungs, which twin sponges are squeezed toward the trunk of the windpipe.

The larynx, too, assumes a posture, its little muscles squeezing to hold open the glottic chink at the top of the trachea to let out the smoke. Aah . . . and out it comes, now a slow-blown wisp, now a fat cloud. It rises about the face. That which was a moment before deep within pours to the out-of-doors, the soul come punctually visible. See it diffuse, coiling fainter and fainter into the general atmosphere. Here is proof—one needs no more—you exist, are *here*, because smoke, that gaseous testimony, is *there*.

One *is*. This smoke is the ultimate assurance.

Here I am, I say to myself . . . and take another puff. It's me.

ABORTION

Horror, like bacteria, is everywhere. It blankets the earth, endlessly lapping to find that one unguarded entryway. As though narcotized, we walk beneath, upon, through it. Carelessly we touch the familiar infected linen, eat from the universal dish; we disdain isolation. We are like the newborn that carry immunity from their mothers' wombs. Exteriorized, we are wrapped in impermeable membranes that cannot be seen. Then one day, the defense is gone. And we awaken to horror.

In our city, garbage is collected early in the morning. Sometimes the bang of the cans and the grind of the truck awaken us before our time. We are resentful, mutter into our pillows, then go back to sleep. On the morning of August 6, 1975, the people of 73rd Street near Woodside Avenue do just that. When at last they rise from their beds, dress, eat breakfast and leave their houses for work, they have forgotten, if they had ever known, that the garbage truck had passed earlier that morning. The event has slipped into unmemory, like a dream.

They close their doors and descend to the pavement. It is midsummer. You measure the climate, decide how you feel in relation to the heat and the humidity. You walk toward the bus stop. Others, your neighbors, are waiting there. It is all so familiar. All at once you step on something soft. You feel it with your foot. Even through your shoe you have the sense of something unusual, something marked by a special "give." It is a foreignness upon the pavement. Instinct pulls your foot away in an awkward little movement. You look down, and you see . . . a tiny naked body, its arms and legs flung apart, its head thrown back, its mouth agape, its face serious. A bird, you think, fallen from its nest. But there is no nest here on 73rd Street, no bird so big. It is rubber, then. A model, a . . . joke. Yes, that's it, a joke. And you bend to see. Because you must. And it is no joke. Such a gray softness can be but one thing. It is a baby, and dead. You cover your mouth, your eyes. You are fixed. Horror has found its chink and crawled in, and you will never be the same as you were. Years later you will step from a sidewalk to a lawn, and you will start at its softness, and think of that upon which you have just trod.

Now you look about; another man has seen it too. "My God," he whispers. Others come, people you have seen every day for years, and you hear them speak with strangely altered voices. "Look," they say, "it's a baby." There is a cry. "Here's another!" and "Another!" and "Another!" And you follow with your gaze the index fingers of your friends pointing from the huddle where you cluster. Yes, it is true! There *are* more of these . . . little carcasses upon the street. And for a moment you look up to see if all the unbaptized sinless are falling from Limbo.

Now the street is filling with people. There are police. They know what to do. They rope off the area, then stand guard over the enclosed space. They are controlled, methodical, these young policemen. Servants, they do not reveal themselves to their public master; it would not be seemly. Yet I do see their pallor and the sweat that breaks upon the face of one, the way another bites the lining of his cheek and holds it thus. Ambulance attendants scoop up the bodies. They scan the street; none must be overlooked. What they place upon the litter amounts to little more than a dozen pounds of human flesh. They raise the litter, and slide it home inside the ambulance, and they drive away. You and your neighbors stand about in the street which is become for you a battlefield from which the newly slain have at last been bagged and tagged and dragged away. *But what shrapnel is this? By what explosion flung, these fragments that sink into the brain and fester there?* Whatever smell there is in this place becomes for you the stench of death. The people of 73rd Street do not then speak to each other. It is too soon for outrage, too late for blindness. It is the time of unresisted horror.

Later, at the police station, the investigation is brisk, conclusive. It is the hospital director speaking: ". . . fetuses accidentally got mixed up with the hospital rubbish . . . were picked up at approximately eight fifteen A.M. by a sanitation truck. Somehow, the plastic lab bag, labeled HAZARDOUS MATERIAL, fell off the back of the truck and broke open. No, it is not known how the fetuses got in the orange plastic bag labeled HAZARDOUS MATERIAL. It is a freak accident." The hospital director wants you to know that it is not an everyday occurrence. Once in a lifetime, he says. But you have seen it, and what are his words to you now?

He grows affable, familiar, tells you that, by mistake, the fetuses got mixed up with the other debris. (Yes, he says *other*; he says *debris*.) He has spent the entire day, he says, trying to figure out how it happened. He wants you to know that. Somehow it matters to him. He goes on:

Aborted fetuses that weigh one pound or less are incinerated. Those weighing over one pound are buried at a city cemetery. He says this. Now you see. It *is* orderly. It *is* sensible. The world is *not* mad. This is still a civilized society.

There is no more. You turn to leave. Outside on the street, men are talking things over, reassuring each other that the right thing is being done. But just this once, you know it isn't. You saw, and you know.

And you know, too, that the Street of the Dead Fetuses will be wherever you go. You are part of its history now, its legend. It has laid claim upon you so that you cannot entirely leave it—not ever.

I am a surgeon. I do not shrink from the particularities of sick flesh. Escaping blood, all the outpourings of disease—phlegm, pus, vomitus, even those occult meaty tumors that terrify—I see as blood, disease, phlegm, and so on. I touch them to destroy them. But I do not make symbols of them. I have seen, and I am used to seeing. Yet there are paths within the body that I have not taken, penetralia where I do not go. Nor is it lack of technique, limitation of knowledge that forbids me these ways.

It is the western wing of the fourth floor of a great university hospital. An abortion is about to take place. I am present because I asked to be present. I wanted to see what I had never seen.

The patient is Jamaican. She lies on the table submissively, and now and then she smiles at one of the nurses as though acknowledging a secret.

A nurse draws down the sheet, lays bare the abdomen. The belly mounds gently in the twenty-fourth week of pregnancy. The chief surgeon paints it with a sponge soaked in red antiseptic. He does this three times, each time a fresh sponge. He covers the area with a sterile sheet, an aperture in its center. He is a kindly man who teaches as he works, who pauses to reassure the woman.

He begins.

A little pinprick, he says to the woman.

He inserts the point of a tiny needle at the midline of the lower portion of her abdomen, on the downslope. He infiltrates local anesthetic into the skin, where it forms a small white bubble.

The woman grimaces.

That is all you will feel, the doctor says. Except for a little pressure. But no more pain.

She smiles again. She seems to relax. She settles comfortably on the table. The worst is over.

The doctor selects a three-and-one-half-inch needle bearing a central stylet. He places the point at the site of the previous injection. He aims it straight up and down, perpendicular. Next he takes hold of her abdomen with his left hand, palming the womb, steadying it. He thrusts with his right hand. The needle sinks into the abdominal wall.

Oh, says the woman quietly.

But I guess it is not pain that she feels. It is more a recognition that the deed is being done.

Another thrust and he has speared the uterus.

We are in, he says.

He has felt the muscular wall of the organ gripping the shaft of his needle. A further slight pressure on the needle advances it a bit more. He takes his left hand from the woman's abdomen. He retracts the filament of the stylet from the barrel of the needle. A small geyser of pale yellow fluid erupts.

We are in the right place, says the doctor. Are you feeling any pain? he asks.

She smiles, shakes her head. She gazes at the ceiling.

In the room we are six: two physicians, two nurses, the patient, and me. The participants are busy, very attentive. I am not at all busy—but I am no less attentive. I want to see.

I see something! It is unexpected, utterly unexpected, like a disturbance in the earth, a tumultuous jarring. I see a movement—a small one. But I have seen it.

And then I see it again. And now I see that it is the hub

of the needle in the woman's belly that has jerked. First to one side. Then to the other side. Once more it wobbles, is *tugged*, like a fishing line nibbled by a sunfish.

Again! And I *know!*

It is the *fetus* that worries thus. It is the fetus struggling against the needle. Struggling? How can that be? I think: *that cannot be.* I think: the fetus feels no pain, cannot feel fear, has no *motivation*. It is merely reflex.

I point to the needle.

It is a reflex, says the doctor.

By the end of the fifth month, the fetus weighs about one pound, is about twelve inches long. Hair is on the head. There are eyebrows, eyelashes. Pale pink nipples show on the chest. Nails are present, at the fingertips, at the toes.

At the beginning of the sixth month, the fetus can cry, can suck, can make a fist. He kicks, he punches. The mother can feel this, can *see* this. His eyelids, until now closed, can open. He may look up, down, sideways. His grip is very strong. He could support his weight by holding with one hand.

A reflex, the doctor says.

I hear him. But I saw something in that mass of cells *understand* that it must bob and butt. And I see it again! I have an impulse to shove to the table—it is just a step— seize that needle, pull it out.

We are not six, I think. We are *seven*.

Something strangles *there*. An effort, its effort, binds me to it.

I do not shove to the table. I take no little step. It would be . . . well, madness. Everyone here wants the needle where it is. Six do. No, *five* do.

I close my eyes. I see the inside of the uterus. It is bathed in ruby gloom. I see the creature curled upon itself. Its knees are flexed. Its head is bent upon its chest. It is in fluid and gently rocks to the rhythm of the distant heartbeat.

It resembles . . . a sleeping infant.

Its place is entered by something. It is sudden. A point coming. A needle!

A spike of *daylight* pierces the chamber. Now the light is extinguished. The needle comes closer in the pool. The point grazes the thigh, and I stir. Perhaps I wake from dozing. The light is there again. I twist and straighten. My arms and legs *push*. My hand finds the shaft—grabs! I *grab*. I bend the needle this way and that. The point probes, touches on my belly. My mouth opens. Could I cry out? All is a commotion and a churning. There is a presence in the pool. An activity! The pool colors, reddens, darkens.

I open my eyes to see the doctor feeding a small plastic tube through the barrel of the needle into the uterus. Drops of pink fluid overrun the rim and spill onto the sheet. He withdraws the needle from around the plastic tubing. Now only the little tube protrudes from the woman's body. A nurse hands the physician a syringe loaded with a colorless liquid. He attaches it to the end of the tubing and injects it.

Prostaglandin, he says.

Ah well, prostaglandin—a substance found normally in the body. When given in concentrated dosage, it throws the uterus into vigorous contraction. In eight to twelve hours, the woman will expel the fetus.

The doctor detaches the syringe but does not remove the tubing.

In case we must do it over, he says.

He takes away the sheet. He places gauze pads over the tubing. Over all this he applies adhesive tape.

I know. We cannot feed the great numbers. There is no

more room. I know, I know. It is a woman's right to refuse
the risk, to decline the pain of childbirth. And an unwanted
child is a very great burden. An unwanted child is a burden
to himself. I know.

And yet . . . there is the flick of that needle. I *saw* it. I
saw . . . I *felt*—in that room, a pace away, life prodded,
life fending off. I saw life avulsed—swept by flood,
blackening—then *out*.

There, says the doctor. It's all over. It wasn't too bad,
was it? he says to the woman.

She smiles. It is all over. Oh, yes.

And who would care to imagine that from a moist and
dark commencement six months before there would ripen
the cluster and globule, the sprout and pouch of man?

And who would care to imagine that trapped within the
laked pearl and a dowry of yoke would lie the earliest stuff
of dream and memory?

It is a persona carried here as well as a person, I think. I
think it is a signed piece, engraved with a hieroglyph of
human genes.

I did not think this until I saw. The flick. The fending
off.

Later, in the corridor, the doctor explains that the law
does not permit abortion beyond the twenty-fourth week.
That is when the fetus may be viable, he says. We stand
together for a moment, and he tells of an abortion in which
the fetus *cried* after it was passed.

What did you do? I ask him.

There was nothing *to* do but let it live, he says. It did
very well, he says. A case of mistaken dates.

THE TWELVE SPHERES

One has it on good authority that the same ills that flesh is heir to in the twentieth century abounded in the Ice Age. In the cave of Trois Frères, in the foothills of the French Pyrenees, for instance, there is painted upon the wall a representation of the typical family doctor of 17,000 years ago. He is wearing a mask in the form of a bison's head, surmounted with bison's horns. He is clearly engaged in the practice of medicine, much as I in my surgeon's cap, mask, and rubber gloves. My instruments of stainless steel replace the flint and obsidian with which he worked. Any further comparison between us would be odious indeed, as it might reveal that much of the romance, if not the art, has gone out of medicine.

There is reason to believe that ill health has existed as long as life itself. Bacteria that exist today have been found fossilized in Cambrian rock layers of 500 million years ago. Parasites that infest us crept into our ancestors. Their preserved remains are 350 million years old. In the fragments of earliest man we have evidence of tumors, dental caries, and joint diseases. One suspects that the reason Neanderthal man did not stand wholly erect was that he was severely afflicted with arthritis, doubtless the result of dwelling in damp caves—a disease for which there is no more effective remedy today than was available to him, poor fellow, who had to hobble in and out of holes in the ground, fend off bears, and procreate painfully on stone floors.

See him, then, Old Doctor Bison, galumphing around the unconscious body of his patient, whose dented skull bears testimony to a blow received in combat or in a fall from a tree. When the demons have been properly frightened away, he performs what remains among the most subtle and dangerous of our operations—trepanning of the skull. There he squats, his back braced against a tree trunk, the patient's head firmly held between his knees. He selects a sharp-edged stone or fleam and makes an incision in the scalp, then bores into and through the bone. Such a stone, if expertly used, can penetrate the human skull in five minutes. He exchanges the dull stone for a new sharp one and bores another hole adjacent to the first, and so on until a complete circle of holes is made. These holes are joined, and the disk of bone is lifted out. There follows a gush of blood and clot, relieving the pressure on the underlying brain. Splinters of loose bone are picked out, and the hole is covered with leaves and mud. Holding aloft the circle of bone, the doctor dances once again, howling and threatening the evil spirits. Soon the labored breathing of the patient subsides into slow, even drafts. He opens his eyes and groans. The doctor stares down at his patient; a surge of great happiness sweeps him. I know, I have felt it myself. Across the ages we are united in a handclasp of congratulations and mutual respect.

What a glorious enterprise was his! Alone, beneath the open sky, no team of consultants, assistants, and nurses milling about to give encouragement or assuage guilt ("You did the best you could"). No vans full of equipment, no oxygen or blood transfusions. Only his crafty hands, sharp stones, and compassion for his injured tribesman. One thrills at his performance.

Testimony to the success of his surgery has been found all over Europe and Asia, where skulls of primitive man have been picked up, many with round holes at the top. The astonishing, humbling fact is that a large number of these holes have smooth, round, well-healed edges, proof of the long-term survival of these patients. They lived long enough to heal the opening in their bone. A good long time! Such skulls have been dredged up from the bottom of the Thames not a mile from where the great English brain surgeons practice today.

In tracing the origins of medicine—a risky exercise, to be sure—one cannot refrain from bandying about three ancient Chinese names. They intrigue by the music of their syllables alone. Spoken aloud, they evoke Chinese temples, bronze gongs, the crackle of altar flames, the spirits of ancestors. They are not unlike magical words that open the gates to enlightenment. The first of these is Fu Hsi, who lived about 5,000 years ago. It is said that he was born after an immaculate conception and twelve years of gestation. Presumably, he spent this time gathering data uninterrupted by all the distractions of extrauterine life. When he finally emerged it was with the trigrams of the *I Ching*, or *Book of Changes*, ready to set down the principles of medical philosophy.

All nature, wrote Fu Hsi, is composed of two opposing cosmic forces, the yin and the yang. The yin is female, soft, receptive, dark, empty. The yang is male, illuminating, creative, firm, constructive. Yin is the earth, yang the heavens. Yin is cold, darkness, disease, and death. Yang is warmth, light, strength, health, and life. Each man is a universe in miniature, composed of and reacting to the interplay of the yin and yang within him. So each organ, each cell. If they are in balance, harmony and health prevail; if not, discord and disease. The religion of Taoism, later founded by Lao-tzu, was based on these principles.

One is struck by the uncanny reasonableness of such a philosophy of balanced and opposing forces. The great bulk of modern medical knowledge of the past thirty years deals with the existence of action and reaction within the body. For example, one is stimulated to take one's next breath by the momentary rise in the level of carbon dioxide following exhalation. This prods the breathing center of the brain to send a message to the lungs to get going, draw in oxygen. The thyroid gland releases its hormone under a system of checks and balances that either stimulates or suppresses the outflow depending on the amount that is already present. The list of such beautiful antagonisms is endless.

The second great name in Chinese medical history is Shen Nung, of a couple of thousand years B.C. Conceived by a princess under the influence of a heavenly dragon, he lived to become the Fire Emperor. He fashioned timbers into plows, taught the people the art of husbandry, and discovered the curative powers of plants. Like Mithridates, King of Pontus, Shen Nung achieved his most deserved reputation in the art of taking poisons. He is said to have tasted seventy different kinds of poison in a single day, and survived to establish the art of medicine. His cast-iron stomach should be our holiest of relics. Four and a half millennia later, John Hunter, an English doctor, proved the infectious nature of syphilis by inoculating his own penis with the scrapings of someone else's chancre. He died of this enthusiasm, and so became the blessed martyr of several ancient professions.

Huang Ti is the third and last of the immaculately conceived founders of medicine. He visited the immortals and received from them the "nineteen gold and silver prescriptions" and the "nine-gourd powder." The goddesses Scarlet and White taught him to interpret the pulse and inspired him to invent the nine acupuncture needles. He set up a stove to prepare his medicines, and thousands of tigers and leopards came to tend the fire for him. When he died at the age of 111, a yellow dragon descended and carried him away. By all standards Huang Ti enjoyed a more fanciful and variegated career than any physician extant with the possible exceptions of Christiaan Barnard and Denton Cooley.

Huang Ti had many followers, not the least of whom was Ma Shih-Huang, the father of veterinary medicine. He was expert in treating horses. Once it happened that a dragon with drooping ears and gaping cold mouth came to him for treatment. He punctured the beast's lips and administered a decoction of licorice, whereupon the dragon's ears rose and bristled, and a satisfying jet of smoke was ejaculated from its mouth. Thereafter many dragons suffering from cold mouth or soft scale came to him, and he cured them all.

Because of the prevalence of ancestor worship in ancient China, autopsy and dissection of the body were forbidden. This taboo remains widespread throughout the world today, even among the most sophisticated of cultures. How often I have been told by the next of kin, when asking permission for an autopsy, "I don't believe in it. It's wrong to cut somebody up like that. He's suffered enough." It was this belief that caused the greatest divergence between the developing paths of Chinese and Western medicine.

Perhaps another reason for the failure of surgery to thrive in China was the traditional disdain of the Chinese doctors for manual labor. This was not strictly a local feeling. For centuries European medicine dwelt in the academy, while surgery was performed in the barbershop. Even today, internists tend to sniff a bit when a surgeon draws nigh. We are held to be generally oafish and bombastic technicians. *They* will do the thinking.

The earliest impulse of our own priest-physicians was to open the body and peer at what lay hidden there, at first with religious awe, later with true objective curiosity. This was to be no rummaging helter-skelter among the viscera but a science sprung out of a need to know and a sense of the beauty of the body. Witness the anatomical drawings of Vesalius and Leonardo da Vinci. The very word *abdomen* is an archaic term whose exact origin cannot be found, but which is thought to come from the ancient Greek word for *hidden* or *occult*. Forbidden this study, Chinese medicine developed into an investigation of the healing powers of herbs, trees, flowers, and other plants, as well as the extracts of lower forms of animal life. It was China, let us never forget, that gave us syrup of deer antler as an aphrodisiac. Any list of the drugs used by the ancient Chinese doctors, for many of which there is ample historical if not laboratory evidence of efficacy, leaves the entire Western world of medicine open to accusations of negligence and haughtiness.

Chinese medicine is not to be judged by the magic and superstition that envelop it, or even by the yin-yang cosmic and animistic beliefs. Rather we must begin to assess Chinese medicine as a system, reflective and philosophical, that considers man's relationship to the vegetable kingdom as well as to his fellows and the other animals. It was in this context that the early physicians began to treat disease with decoctions brewed from herbs, trees, minerals, and animal parts. Thus, they knew that watermelon was useful in the treatment of dropsy, that it increased the volume of urine and decreased swelling. The same paregoric or tincture of opium that is now used throughout the world as a treatment for diarrhea, as well as being rubbed on the gums of teething babies, had the same purposes in China before the Christian era. The most commonly used nasal decongestant, ephedrine, cleared the upper respiratory passages of the ancients and relieved their asthma. If these and many others, then why not at least an equal number of as yet untested herbs and extracts? It is just possible that the happiest outflow from our détente with China will be in the domain of medicine. At least one hitherto unknown drug derived from a Chinese tree purported to have anticancer properties is already under investigation at the National Institutes of Health in Bethesda, Maryland, and Chinese literature even refers to the complete cure of malignant tumors. Whether or not this single medicament will bear Western fruit, it indicates that at last our investigative science is turning, beelike, to the thousand flowers of China. It no longer boggles the Western mind that we may one day be treated with such materia medica as deer-horn velvet for convulsions and anemia, or dried venom of Chinese toads for the common cold. I must confess that something within me yearns to write such prescriptions, apply such unguents. Perhaps it is the desire to regain that immediate sense of man as part of nature, perhaps the joy of confounding pharmacists.

Though surgery was all but nonexistent in ancient China, surgical legend abounds. Witness the tale of the man who had a tumor between his eyes that itched intolerably. The famous Dr. Hua P'o examined it, and said there was a bird in it. When the tumor was opened, sure enough, a canary flew out, and the patient was cured. The appealing poetics of this story are a statement on the independent life of disease, that it flourishes, waxes, and wanes much as do all other living processes. Here, it is a canary released from the body where it was trapped, to fly freely toward some other destiny. A very Chinese idea. We, of course, would like to have seen the canary dead, its little head cut off, its body stomped—take that and that, you dirty bird—which says something about the difference in subtlety between Chinese medical thought and our own.

For thousands of years the two most commonly performed operations in China were castration and the binding of feet, procedures for which there is not a great call today. We have found less immediately painful and more subtle ways to castrate ourselves, and the foot fetishism has been reduced from a national obsession to a somewhat furtive refinement of individuals. Nonetheless, eunuchs held a certain enviable position of power and leisure in Old China, being raised as privileged servants of princes, and it was not at all considered *lèse majesté* for the teen-age son of good family to opt for the soft life in this fashion.

The binding of feet, while not strictly surgical, used what might be loosely construed as reconstructive plastic-surgery techniques. It was altogether a pernicious deed. The toes and bones of the foot were bent under until they touched the heel, the arch bent, and the foot bound tightly in this position. The consequent atrophy and deformity often achieved a foot length of three inches, and made of walking a birdlike trip and hop that was always painful. Chinese men were fascinated by these tiny feet, called them "golden lilies," and loved to play with and sing about them. The ideal foot, wrote the poet Fang Hsien, is fat and elegant. Thin feet are cold, and muscular feet are hard and vulgar. The fatness and softness may be judged by sight and touch, but the elegance is appreciated only by "the eye of the mind." (Mutilation in the name of fashion is not peculiarly Chinese. Consider an American example: the multiplicity of cosmetic operations undergone by both men and women unwilling or unable to accept themselves as they are or as they have become. One thinks of *mammo-plasty*—either augmentation, in which the breasts are made larger, or reduction, in which they are made smaller—and the even more prevalent face-lift. In short, it is a matter not of principle, but of degree. One wonders whether our own descendants will view these procedures as the fruits of surgical skill or as primitive rites.)

All this brings us to that most intriguing holdover from ancient Chinese medical practices, acupuncture. Chinese medicine is not directed toward discovering the causes of

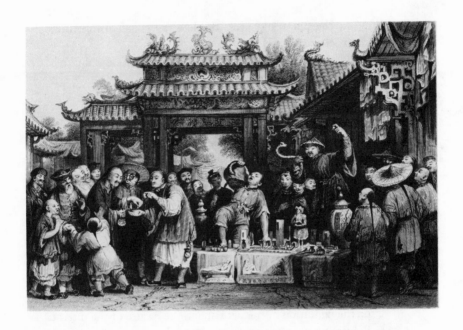

disease, but toward simply studying the phenomena themselves. The best-known example of this is the recognition
of a correspondence between the covering of the body and
its internal contents. In this view, the skin is a screen upon
which the organs are in some way projected, so that stimu-
lating a specific spot on this screen will influence a specific
organ. The route of transmission of this impulse remains
unknown.

After the goddesses Scarlet and White gave the concept
of acupuncture to Huang Ti, he made several needles out
of flint and bone. These needles were of various shapes and
sizes. Originally, 365 points on the body surface which had

a specific relation to the internal organs were used. The early method of acupuncture is given in twelve instructions:

1. Mark the point and press the left thumbnail firmly there to expel the air and blood.
2. Hold the needle in the right hand. The mind should be concentrated and the strength sustained.
3. Warm the needle by holding it in the mouth.
4. Avoid piercing the arteries.
5. During the operation, if the air does not flow freely, gently stroke the surrounding tissues with the fingers.
6. If there is resistance to the entrance of the needle, press along the course of the "channel" with the thumbnail.
7. The needle should be withdrawn very slowly, the patient taking three deep breaths during the process.
8. In puncturing, the needle should be twisted or screwed in to the required depth.
9. Rotate the needle to the right or to the left according to the result desired.
10. The length of time that the needle remains *in situ* depends on the condition of the patient and the nature of the disease.
11. Before drawing out the needle, shake it several times so as to relieve the tension.
12. Press the left thumb over the spot after the needle has been pulled out, in order to stop bleeding and prevent air from getting in.

From this simple and rather pedestrian set of instructions, it is obvious that the art could be practiced by anyone with two hands and a flair for the dramatic. In fact, this is what happened, which may be why acupuncture fell into disrepute and has remained there, except in China itself and in several enclaves of interest in France and England.

Reading accounts of the practice of acupuncture as it has been done in China during the past five hundred years produces an all-encompassing skepticism. Say, for example, that one is in Suifu, a town in the province of Szechuan in western China. The year is 1880. A large crowd has collected in the marketplace. One approaches to find that in the center of the crowd is a Chinese surgeon engaged in the practice of acupuncture. He is wearing a long blue robe soiled by bloodstains, the extrusion of various wounds, and the various leavings of the body.

Spread on the ground near his feet are huge charts and diagrams of the body showing the numerous points of acupuncture and revealing the lines of influence or the meridians along which the needle must be thrust. These charts are as tattered and soiled as their owner, giving the appearance of immense age. The people are impressed by this as by the mystifying nature of the diagrams. The surgeon bends over his charts, poring, tracing a particular line with a stick. His face is weighted with concentration. He is oblivious to the crowd. He straightens, and approaches the first patient, a woman, seated on a bench. Her breathing is heavy and moist. With each inspiration, her nostrils flare to widen the indraft. There is a pallor about her mouth, and the veins of her neck are swollen and full. In the surgeon's hand is a six-inch copper needle, which he runs through his hair six times in order to clean it, then lubricates it in his mouth. A hush falls over the crowd. He selects a point on the right half of the patient's forehead, marks the point with his left thumbnail, and then inserts the needle, twisting it inward to a depth of half an inch. Then he backs off. The patient wears the needle hanging from her forehead with the patience and resignation of a domesticated beast. If it is painful she does not show it. Soon a second needle is passed through her left ear, then a third into the front of her neck. One watches as it throbs in response to the great vessels close to which it lies. A fourth and fifth are applied, and she looks as though she has fallen headlong into a cactus. Before his day's work is done the benches about him will be filled with men, women, and children all pierced by many needles. No part of the body is spared, and each puncture is studiously read in the charts. At sundown, the last needle has been retrieved, and the charts are rolled up. The crowd has long since dispersed. Many developed serious infections. Others hemorrhaged internally, and some died. Who was there to say that the cause of death was not the disease process but the physician himself?

What kept acupuncture alive throughout the centuries was the undeniable fact that vast numbers of patients were relieved of their pain, or could breathe more easily by submitting to the needles.

Dare we, smugly entrenched in the scientific method, ask how, when we do not have the least idea how aspirin relieves headache and decreases fever? Aspirin, the most widely used drug in the world, works—and that's all we know about it.

There has now arisen a whole new race of acupuncturists with great colored charts on their walls. At $50 to $100 a prick they claim to—and *do*—relieve pain, nausea, and cough unresponsive to all the elaborate ministrations of Western medicine. Moreover, and unhappily, they attempt to tell us how it works. Felix Mann, for example, in his book *Acupuncture: The Ancient Chinese Art of Healing and How It Works Scientifically*, invokes the nervous system as the transmitter of the needle stimuli, and he theorizes the existence of the cutaneovisceral reflex.

To prove the existence of such a reflex he cites various experimental works, offering such evidence as the constriction of the blood vessels of the intestine when a beaker of ice is applied to the back. Peristalsis of the intestine is also altered by hot or cold applications to the skin of the upper abdomen. But the fact remains that none of the experimental work examined could stand close scrutiny in an unbiased laboratory. The experiments are simplistic and the results prejudged. Where the whole system of acupuncture falls down is in the attempts to explain it. I would, if anything, prefer to accept it on faith, to receive it as the distillate of 5,000 years of Chinese wisdom that has stood the test of time. Unlike many of my colleagues, I would not insist upon a rigid investigation into cause and effect at this time. It is obviously not forthcoming. We are then faced with the choice of relegating acupuncture to the realm of quackery or entertaining the heresy that there are some things we do not know, of which we have not the least understanding, and before which we can only bow until such time as we shall be enlightened by a shaft of scientific grace.

Any attempt to study the art of acupuncture is threatening to the mental health, and as a physician I strongly advise against it. For those who are making a marginal adjustment as it is, it might be just the thing to tip the balance into madness and overt lunacy. Acupuncture, to use Yul Brynner's exasperated expression in *The King and I*, is a puzzlement, and only those who are happy wandering in labyrinths ought to look into it. I myself have tried, believe me, to examine the charts, follow the meridians about the body, identify the points with some sense of order, and am only now recovering my composure after a prolonged indisposition.

I would much prefer to study the Chinese myth of creation and to comtemplate its similarity to our own. In the beginning was P'an Ku, the horned dwarf. Heaven was his father; Earth his mother. Dressed in an apron of leaves and carrying a mallet and chisel, he pounded and chipped the rude masses of matter into shape. He breathed, and the wind arose. By the opening of his eyes, the day began. For eighteen thousand years the Son of Heaven labored to fashion the universe, and when his work was done, he gave up his life, settling into his masterpiece. His head became the mountains, his breath the wind and clouds. Thunder was his voice, the sun his left eye, the moon his right. All the strata of the earth were his veins and muscles. The soil was his very flesh, the rain his sweat, and the lice upon his body became man.

(Now aside from certain details of costume and a tendency toward slowness, it is not an unsurmountable gap between the grand Chinese myth of creation and our own. I am willing to be persuaded that we who insist upon those six days of work, and the seventh of rest, are unrealistic and quite carried away by our fervor.) The lousy origin of the human species may offend the sensibilities of many, still it is a sweet and appealing idea that humbles as it elevates all creatures great and small.

IV
DOWN FROM TROY

DOWN FROM TROY

My father practiced medicine in Troy, whose ruins lay tumbled midway on the old via dolorosa from New York to Montreal. Since he was born in the former, and had graduated from McGill Medical School in the latter in 1924, he must have regarded Troy as a reasonable geographical compromise. More likely, he and my mother and the old Hudson had run out of gas on the way south and, either from inertia or in a flash of impulsiveness, had decided to flop where they were. For some years Mother had attracted attention over a six-block spread of St. Urbain Street in Montreal by the small trilly soprano with which she had rendered "Pale Hands I Loved Beside the Shalimar" and "What Are the Wild Waves Saying?" This before hushed clusters of illegal immigrants from eastern Europe who did not know Kashmir from Kracow. Whatever the reason, their decision to settle in Troy seems, in retrospect, to have been a morose concession to stick with the lower class and hope for the best.

It seems only innocence, which I find endearing, that could have led them to view this moribund town as the land of milk and honey. By the time my brother Billy and I had finished our first decade of life, Troy had been out of these staples for an equal period of time. Troy, in the nine-

teen thirties, was a cobblestoned heaven from across the
Irish Sea—ninety percent Irish and one hundred percent
underprivileged, a city afflicted with "failure to thrive," the
population declining by a few hundred each year. The
sound in the streets each evening was not the warm respiration of urban life, but an endless agonal gasp of a town that
was being garotted by its major industry—the manufacture
of collars. Long after the world of fashion had pronounced
the passing of the collar as an article of apparel, and the
board of health had condemned collars as a major cause of
boils, we went right on manufacturing them, thousands
each month, with truly touching zeal.

Still, Father continued to administer injections of bee
venom to the local arthritics, and diathermy treatments to
anyone with lumbago who would lie still long enough, and
who was not put off by the terrifying electrical inadequacy
of his antique apparatus. This plus the lancing of the innumerable boils to which we were occupationally prone, and
the delivery of a hundred or so scrawny new Trojans each
year, made up the bulk of his professional activities. In no
way do I mean to denigrate him as a physician. On the
contrary, I am convinced that when the lifetime of "good"
done by each of us has been toted up, his will exceed mine
thrice times thrice. He was a compassionate man who loved
his patients as they loved him, and that is probably most
essential in the practice of medicine.

We lived on the second floor of an elderly infirm brown-
stone at 45 Second Street. Father's office was on the first
floor, a fact somewhat diffidently announced to the world
by a rectangle of milk glass in one of the two front windows. "J. L. Selzer, M.D., C.M.," it read, and a companion
piece in the other window: "Office Hours 1–3, 6–8." "No
Appointments" was added in small print at the bottom. It
was that "No Appointments" that spoke volumes about the
state of health of his practice. Those letters "M.D., C.M."
were the only truly romantic things in our life. Especially

"C.M.," which I found out later meant Master of Chirurgie. Such a Latinism, even abbreviated in a place like Troy, rather set one aside from the general populace.

That our living quarters were above the office might at first glance be considered eminently convenient. Actually, it was an arrangement quite deleterious to the psychological development of Billy and me. It was understood by us from the days of our swaddling clothes and bunting that there was to be no noise made between one and three, and six and eight, every day save Sunday. The patients came first, and we were to be neither seen nor heard, which is one step further than even the Victorian adage decreed. Billy and I learned to converse in hoarse whispers and to convey oceans of intent by the smallest of facial twitches.

Our house on Second Street was undistinguished except for a certain back room in the cellar, which beckoned eerily to my brother and me.

No one ever went down there. The only set of stairs had long since given up all pretensions to an architecture for descent or elevation, and hung gaptoothed and undulating, lacking but a single unearthly laugh to send them crumpling to the ground. Billy and I had been forbidden to trespass in a way that clearly meant that violation of the proscribed premises was in no wise to be leniently grouped with inferior table manners, but was right up there with masturbation and painting Grandpa's dentures with the watercolors, each tooth a different pastel.

As Eve was drawn to the gonadal apples of her serpent, as Leda to her "feathered glory," so were my brother and I pulled by some base and ancient allure to the dank fetor of that cellar room, as though it were the sunken gray womb of Earth itself. We were two Orphei descending, and no lyre to pluck whose notes would tame that darkness, no Eurydice waiting to embolden us by her pallor. Once that door to the back stairs had closed behind us, we had only the quest for adventure, the drive toward danger that has characterized both our greatest explorers and our most gifted psychopaths.

Strategy decreed that we should descend one at a time. Our combined weight would surely overtax the ruin strung before us. Billy, who was thirteen months older, and thus the bearer of the flashlight, was to go first. I to await his call when he had reached the bottom. I waited with fierce yearning, a painful throbbing in my chest for what seemed to me eons of eerie time. At last the soft call, "Come." The whisper floated upward like a last exhalation. It was a beckoning, the call of a Siren, at once terrifying and irresistible. "Me, come?" I thought for one brief instant, and then . . . went. Step after step, scrabbling as a Sherpa descending Everest, leaning upon the darkness, prehending the boards with my toes, exhorting my skin to a stickiness the better to adhere to whatever solid matter might materialize. I went, urged by that mixture of death-wish and bravado that must spur those men who charm snakes or dine on wild mushrooms. The susurration of "ssshes" from my brother and the twinkling of his little light seemed a star away. Lower and lower I swung from cobweb to cobweb as though they were ropy vines.

All at once, a hand reached from out that night and grasped my arm. It was as though my chest had suddenly sprung open from chin to navel, and I felt my unprisoned heart bound from its cage. I swear I could see it hovering in the air, all red and glowing, exteriorized, like St. Catherine of Siena's when she prayed, and held hers out to Jesus. It was not prayer, nor love, nor truth that made me whole again. It was when I could see that it was Billy who grabbed me and not the ghost of 45 Second Street. I took the hand held out to me and moored myself to it. Billy played the beam of light in slow circles about the room. There were shelves on the wall lined with old bottles stoppered with corks, each one partially full of a murky liquid. In one corner leaned a pickaxe. So long had it stood that one of its points had settled into the earthen floor like a galleon embedded in the bottom of the ocean. The walls were of moldy brick between which oozed spectral little plants, grayish white in color, that felt like cold swollen worms. Never having seen the light of day, they had long since given up their craving for chlorophyll or any other of the good things of the out-of-doors, much as certain religious who renounce the world and, after a novitiate of active self-denial, are strangely content. A psoriatic rash of lichen scabbed these bricks and gave off a sour-smelling exudate.

"What's that?" I pointed our fused appendages toward a concentrate of blackness mounding against a wall.

"Let's see," said Billy.

"It looks like a chest," I offered.

"It *is* a chest," said Billy. A pirate's chest! And indeed, our fully dilated pupils made out the rolling hump of the lid, the rusted hinges, the moldering wood.

"What do you suppose is in it?" For a long time we stood before the chest, immobile as deer sniffing danger in the tall grass, and all the while a hurricane of possibility made wreakage of our logic. Was it gold? Rubies? Ivory? Was it some scented smoke that, once unleashed, would grant us dreadful wishes, demand unspeakable acts?

"I wonder if we can open it," said Billy and shook off my hand which had all but grown to his.

"Here, you take the flashlight, and hold it on the lock," he said. Even then I was consumed with resentment that two people from the same womb slipped, and graced or burdened with the identical heritage, should vary so profoundly in the matter of courage. Of the two teeth sown, one was a dragon's, the other that of a rabbit. The beam of light trembled on the lock. With a kind of frenzy I watched his fingers swim in and out of the pale shaft like hooded white minnows.

"Hold still," he hissed. I held, but not still.

"It's not locked," came the words. "It's open! Help me lift the lid."

Together we sank our fingertips into the crack beneath the lid, and lifted until it was resting against the wall behind.

The first things we saw were the skulls resting on top of the other bones, side by side, blinking in the light. They seemed to be up to their chins in bones—leg, arm, finger, and back, arranged in no order but lying athwart each other in terrible disarray. How long had they dwelt there, those two, before we had surprised them? Who were they?

"God," whispered Billy. I noted with some satisfaction that even his voice shook as the limits of his bravery were overcome.

"I dare you to touch one," said Billy.

"I double dare *you*," I replied.

"Double dares go first," he said with absolute finality.

It was true. Such were the rules of the game. Double dares did go first. In my distraction I had slipped into the kind of superfluousness of expression that was to plague and embarrass me all the days of my life. Whether it was some long forgotten devotion to the concept of The Game, whether I had gone this far and thus could somehow go a little farther, or whether it was the kind of hooded defiance that one imagines summoning opposite a firing squad, I reached out one index finger and touched, ever so lightly, one of the skulls in the center of the forehead. With a tiny clatter, it fell backward on its bed of bones, and lay there staring upward. If my years be Methuselan, I shall never forget the dry dustiness, the coolness, the hardness of that touch. Nor shall the echo of that faint clatter ever cease to reverberate in my mind.

That our father had murdered two persons and concealed their remains in the cellar was instantly apparent to us both. We stared alternately at the bones and at each other, our heads swiveling in little arcs of wild surmise.

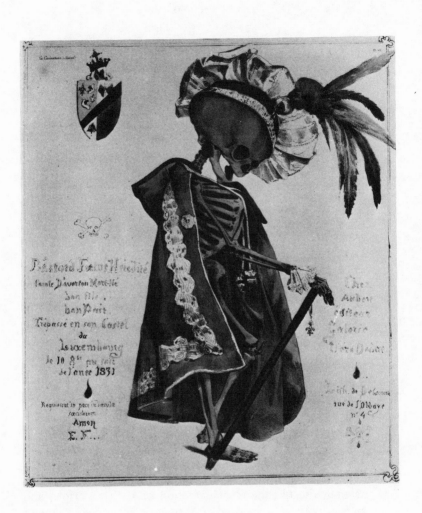

"It was two patients," said Billy. "Probably stung 'em with too much bee venom or electrocuted 'em with that diathermy machine. He didn't dare tell, so he stuck 'em down here. Oh my God."

"I bet it was enemies," I said, "jealous rivals, come to kill him in the dead of night but he got 'em first." This was clearly absurd, for if there was one thing that our father did not have, it was a rival. Only lunatics vie for failure.

"I bet he hasn't told Ma. She'd kill him. We're the only ones who know."

Locking our icy fingers, we took upon ourselves the bloody sleeves of conspiracy.

"I'll never tell a soul. Don't you either, or they'll come and take him away." It was so resolved.

We lowered the lid of the chest and mounted that staircase from Hell, and all the while a cold stream of panic washed over the two small pebbles that were our hearts. Our coming of age had nothing to do with the development of secondary sex characteristics, the rising of sap, or the ripening of fruit, in preparation for which we had spent hours committing to memory the diagrams of the female pudenda in Gray's *Anatomy* and Williams' *Obstetrics*. For Billy and me, "passage" had to do only with our secret. For days we haunted the house like spectres, speaking in whispers, taking to our beds early in the evening, only to lie awake for hours hoarsely reliving the descent into the cellar, conjecturing anew on the identity of the two bodies, arguing the likelihood of detection of Father's crime, and ending with an exhausted reaffirmation of our covenant of silence.

The most awkward moments were at the dinner table when Father was carving a chicken. In thrall to our preoccupation, Billy and I would stare at him, his hands engaged in the dismemberment. We were scarcely able to breathe, much less to express preference for white or dark meat. Father took inordinate pride in his carving, doubtless a holdover from the lancing of all those boils. He would hone the bone-handled blade on its rasp with the kind of surgical savor observed among Edwardian butlery. For him it was a ritual, to be performed slowly and with elegance. There was to be a building up of culinary suspense, culminating in that delicious first mouthful. For my brother and me. it became a practice such as might be witnessed at a Black Mass.

Days went by, weeks heavy with depression and worry. Like Troy itself, we failed to thrive, lost weight, became spidery and full of sighs. No call to baseball lot or park was heeded. Nor could we bear to listen to our favorite radio program, *Inner Sanctum*. The sound of that creaking door was enough to pry loose our desperate abraded fingertips from the cliff edge of reason.

As time went on, so great was our horror it seemed that in some subliminal way, far below the threshold of consciousness, those two skeletons had become us, that by some strange inconsistency of time, Billy and I had come face to face with our own mortal remains. It was no less than the prophetic evidence of our own violent and grisly demises to come.

At last there came the day, as we must have known it would, when the limits of endurance were reached. It was Sunday dinner, and *he* was carving. Billy and I watched, sick with a mixture of pity and contempt. Father had just neatly separated a drumstick from the carcass when, with sudden resolution, he laid down the knife and rose from his chair at the head of the table. For a long moment he did not speak, but gazed first at Billy, then me. At last he spoke.

"All right," he said, "out with it. For weeks you've been slinking around here like a pair of sick alley cats. And staring. What, in God's name, are you staring at all the time? If you do not tell me at once, I shall give you, right now, the thrashing that you so richly deserve."

It was Billy who spoke, his voice low, sepulchral.

"We know," he said.

"Yes," I echoed. "We know."

"Oh," said Father. "You know, then."

We nodded. He sat down quickly, we supposed to keep himself from falling to the floor, then looked fixedly at the disarticulated chicken with what seemed to us ineffable sorrow.

"What," he said at last, in a hushed tone, "what do you know?"

A flood of relief! At last we were free to acknowledge our awful fact, to share it with him, to join him as beloved accessories. A torrent of words burbled from our mouths.

"We know all about the chest in the cellar, and the bones. We saw it. There were two, the heads side by side. I touched it, but we won't tell a soul. We swear it. Honest to God, we won't."

A shock of recognition flitted across his face, as though his worst fears had been realized. In a moment it was gone.

"So you know, then," he said sadly. "Now you know everything."

A sense of impending doom settled over the dinner table. Creases of woe appeared suddenly upon Father's brow. He seemed to shrivel into great age before our very eyes.

"You . . . you won't tell anyone?" The sound of that voice, heretofore so stern and masterful, now quavering weakly, dripping with beseechment, brought us running to him, tears streaming from our eyes, to assure him that his secret was safe with us forever. I, for one, would have undergone torture to the death, and still maintained my silence.

"Thank you," murmured Father, and his hands covered his fallen face. After a few minutes he appeared to recover himself at the cost of great effort.

"And now," he said, "I think it is time for us to eat our dinner."

Never was food consumed with such appetite.

It was three weeks later that I overheard Father telling Uncle Henry the story of how we found the bones of his old medical school skeletons, and of how we thought he had killed two people, and of what happened at the dinner table, and they both laughed like hell for an obscenely long time.

To achieve failure in Troy in 1934 was not beyond the grasp of most men. Doctors, lawyers, coopers, and carpenters alike sucked the dry stones of poverty. Only the clergy were astir, harrying sin like belly-pinched wolves, intoning, drawing for us the Hereafter as Wonderland. Were I now by some sleight-of-time able to return to Troy and to that age, I would go as a clown, to tumble and take pratfalls, to heal all my dear countrymen with antic and with sweet imposture.

In such a clutch of circumstance some men stole, others drank; still others lay down for dying. Father did none of these, but quietened into dreaming. Or was it madness? But I malign the man. He did no raving in the dead of night. Nor did he violate the oath of Hippocrates with secret abortion, that unspeakable act of the day. Instead, he went furtive—through his empty waiting room, to his desk—and took up his pen to write *fiction*. It was all about a prostitute named Goldie (after her heart) and the sensual brooding doctor who falls in love with her, all the while struggling with his atheism. In the end she gives him up, thereby restoring his faith. It is one of my lifelong regrets that the manuscript has not been preserved. Now that I too have been reduced to the anguish of writing fiction, it should be my holy scripture, my beacon, and my emblem. As it is, I am a writer unmoored, in search of a heritage, catching at stray ancestors. Ah, if only I could weep over *his* metaphors, fondle the pages where his alphabet was spilled.

For three years he wrote. When the novel was done he presented it to Mother. "Keep it away from the children," she said. So Father decided to cure athlete's foot. Of the thirteen years of our acquaintance on earth, the last three were devoted to this project with a singleness of purpose that filial piety insists I call quixotic. Under conditions of secrecy that would rival those veiling Los Alamos, he devised the infamous unguent called Will's Foot Balm after his firstborn son, in the manner of Old Testament patriarchy. Sheer melancholy prevents me from listing the countless combinations of ingredients which he ground in his mortar and pestle, or swirled in his flasks. No witch, cave-bound or forestine, steeped in her cauldron a more romantic stew. It had everything but eye of newt. The final receipt, as I recall it, contained glycerine, rose water, brilliantine, coal tar, sulfur, balsam of Peru, and oil of eucalyptus.

It was the old kitchen stove's finest hour. Pots and pans of Balm sat over its burners day and night, simmering. They required constant stirring, and Father's thin white hairless arms wound in ceaseless circles through the steam. High as prayer it was, this ritual of alchemy. There were the fumes of incense, the bubbling, the drone of hope. As Apostles of the Creed, Billy and I spooned gobbets of Balm into the one-, two-, and three-ounce jars upon which Father had spent his only dollars, while Mother pasted labels and sang "Mighty 'Lak a Rose." We were a happy band of conspirators and, like all fanatics, had fallen in love with our work—the grinding, stirring, boiling, decanting, and filtering of it.

Was it not a holy enterprise to be engaged in easing the footsore of the world? Nor, truth to tell, was the dream of untold riches far from our thoughts. No hidden cell of secret dreamers throbbed with such a hopeful heart. After all, to transform common fungus into coin of the realm was no mean feat.

That we remained poor and that athlete's foot remains the scourge of mankind are (yes, I must) injustices of Fate.

The first seven patients upon whom Will's Foot Balm was smeared developed a relentless and painful exfoliative dermatitis of the toes. Malpractice suits were not yet à la mode. The settlement was more direct. And one day Father returned from his office with a swollen lip and blood at the corners of his mouth. In his hand he carried one of his incisor teeth. To my knowledge Will's Foot Balm was never again applied to living flesh, and whether or not the blight of fungus foot would have been eradicated from the face of the earth remains irretrievably unanswered. Perhaps some other, as yet unborn, alchemist will reconstruct this ancient formula and mix and stir his pots to the wild rhythm of his heart.

The grieving pantry shelves remained stacked with the little white jars. Three-ounce on the bottom, two-ounce in the middle, and the ones on the top, each one a monument to folly, and the whole a terrible graveyard of materia medica. In the end only Mother was able to enter the pantry comfortably. For Father the jars were the mementos of a mistress too recklessly adored. Mother, and Mother alone, could face such a rival. For Billy, as for me, the pantry was a catacomb wherein a third and martyred sibling had been laid. One upon whom we had doted without restraint and who had disappointed us by dying.

It was unlucky Thursday when Father was seized by the heart and hurled to the echoless linoleum, then catapulted to the hospital, room 204. There were voices, Mother's and Billy's.

"Do you think he is suffering?"

There was a long silence during which I heard heavy wet breathing that bubbled up from beneath a surface somewhere.

"It looks to be such a hard time. Oh, I know it is. The tossing."

"No, you mustn't, Billy. He's quieter now. He's easy."

Every second, one drop. Sixty each minute, as precise and alike as tears. It was absurd to tell the time by them, yet it was all the time there was, and for as long as I was able, I gazed at the intravenous fluid dripping from the bottle into Father's arm. At last the drops fused, coalesced into a kind of rain, and I lost track. Then I feared the fluid washing out the redness of the blood, feared that it was leaching Father of his personal brine. Soon he would be as bland and clear as an angel. Once Father opened his eyes, and saw us. He smiled then and formed "Hello there" with his mouth, and I could see the space where one of his teeth was missing.

He was in an oxygen tent, and through the walls his lips were the color of pavement, his nostrils flared like an animal's at bay. All at once, disengaged somehow from his private grapple, he smiled again at me, and raised one hand to wave. It seemed that something as thin and white as a handkerchief had floated up from the bed, then slowly settled back. A little later I was led back into the room to see the body.

"Our Daddy has passed away," said Mother. That was the first time she had ever called him that. I knew at once that this was the formality of death. One took a certain stance. I was told to kiss Father goodbye, which I did with my eyes wide open, entering the oxygen tent, feeling the cold plastic on the back of my neck, and thinking of packaged steak. I bent, and watched the gray meaty face come closer and closer to my own. When I pressed my lips to that dark doughy mouth it was still wet with cold saliva. It was the one kiss I was to remember all my life, whose taste and texture would spring to my lips at any moment without any warning. I never really liked kissing after that, although I have done a lot of it to be congenial.

Two days later, under the sky there was the sound of earth falling on polished walnut. The walls of the grave seemed naked, embarrassingly so. They ought not to have been left exposed like that, I thought, and lifted away my eyes.

"Are you thirteen?" someone asked.

Yes, I nodded, and looked at Mother, wondering what she was thinking, knowing that it couldn't possibly be anything good or happy.

"I hope we can be buried together," she said.

CAR SICKNESS

I sing of cars and passengers. Of those who suffer from car sickness. Would that mankind might earn the largeness of spirit to embrace these pitiful outscourings of the human race, who do but express in unequivocal terms their antipathy toward the automobile. Lacking perhaps the physiological restraint of astronauts, the decorum of hikers, and the delirium of jockeys, with all of whom they share this mutual contempt of cars, the victims of car sickness are shunned like lepers by a society that takes callous pride only in ac and de celeration.

For the greater part of my life I have been among those wretches with what I shall henceforth call mal de voiture, in whom the mere slamming of a car door is enough to bring on the first wamblings of nausea.

Sunday in Troy was a day of retrenchment. About the only thing to do was to take a ride en famille to the country. This was not mere custom; it was rite. Everyone did it, as though it were some elemental thread binding us to our forefathers and our descendants. A ride in the country was healthy; it was restorative; and, at least for me, it was dreadful. How I yearned to be left behind to wander alone the unmoving pavement, the changeless cobblestones of Troy until, come nightfall, I could welcome home the rustic riders serene of heart, steady of stomach. Such a leaving was not meant to be. More, it was considered tantamount to disloyalty by my father and child abandonment by my mother, who, at the mere suggestion, would whiten at the imagined horrors that would surely befall me, left alone and palely loitering. At the very least I would descend to solitary or group vice, touch the dark underside of Trojan life, and be lost forever to the lists of decent people. Perhaps she was right at that. The propensity for such a fall has ever been just beneath my surface, and it is a wise mother who knows her own child.

Thus was all entreaty denied, all supplication ill-received. Fate had decreed that I was to celebrate the Sabbath in my own fashion all over Rensselaer and the adjacent counties of upstate New York. I have vomited in Saratoga, Glens Falls, and Speculator; in French Cohoes as in Dutch Albany; in the pastoral town of Melrose and all along the Mohawk Trail. In every country corner of our land I deposited my unparceled ejecta so that the callowest novice of a hunter could have traced the motorings of our family by my pathetic spoor. Would time stand still, I wondered, and Monday never come were I to fail to carry out this ritual? In the throes of mal de voiture I decided that I had been chosen to suffer for a higher purpose as yet unknown to me, and that when the true meaning of my affliction would be revealed, I would be venerated as, if not the patron saint, at least the martyr of the automobile.

"It's all in your head," said Father.

"Mind over matter," said Mother.

For a time I believed them, and would tell myself stories in a constant murmuring undertone to match the hums of the motor. In one I was a strange sinewy Tartar who returned from riding his horse through fields of flowers, and the sweet smell of the hooves of my steed would cause to swoon the beautiful yellow princess who waited. This story merely hastened the inevitable gastric upheaval. In another I was the Royal Gardener of the Empress Wu of the T'ang dynasty who had petulantly ordered that all the flowers in the Imperial Garden were to bloom on the same day. By virtue of my horticultural genius I was able to bring this about, with the sole exception of the sweet-smelling peony, which refused to bloom, for which revolutionary act I was beheaded. But first I threw up.

Later when I had reached the age of reason I came to know the feeble mutterings of my parents as airy persiflage. It had nothing to do with mind. Ever since, I have looked askance at the hypotheses of psychosomatic medicine. Years later I learned, not without some bitter satisfaction, that my distress was due to the tilting of fluid in my middle ear, that this caused an alteration in my sense of position relative to things outside, leading to reflex nausea and its roadside consummation. The straight unemotional flavor of these scientific words was nothing short of a justification for my existence. With what untrammeled joy did I read that the doughty astronauts suffered motion sickness aboard their mooncraft, and were reduced to mouthing comfort bags. The suffering of our heroes has always made us happy. Alas, even these truths did not set me free.

You have not known true agony until you have struggled to contain an attack of mal de voiture. There is the first skidding shudder of the stomach, the telltale yawn, the gathering of saliva, the fullness of the abdomen that insists that belt and clothing be loosened and held free of the skin—even the slightest contact will speed the internal vortex—the clenching of the teeth, the grim efforts at distraction, the fixing of the gaze straight ahead, and finally the awful knowledge that nothing is going to help. There comes the moment when resolve snaps, and the sour belch of despair fills the car with its rank miasma. Now you grow cold, turn green. You sweat. Soon you will die. And all the while there is the guilt laced with shame that you have,

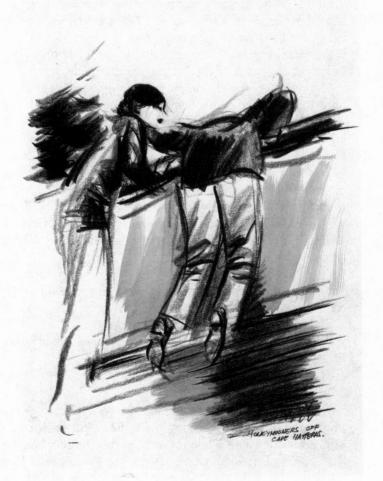

HONEYMOONERS OFF
CAPE HATTERAS.

with cank and with cark, spoiled the ride. You are a killjoy, a blight.

Then comes the whispered command from your lips: "Stop the car." Who would think that such a phrase, barely audible, scarcely more than an exhalation, would bring the demon to an immediate halt? Wordless now you slip from the car to slump against the nearest tree, a rock, the ground, whilst the survivors, torn by their own violent emotions, alternately watch the drama unfold or turn aside to gaze in envy at the happy tourists whizzing by.

Only Father would dismount, heaving himself from behind the wheel to stand behind me, one hand supporting my forehead, the other arm looped about my pelvis, holding me upright. Little beads of disappointment, I supposed, formed and burst in his chest. What comfort could he take in this rancid geyser of a son whose well-being depended upon remaining motionless? O sharper than a serpent's tooth to have a car-sick child! At last, my heart all laden with rue, I was led back in disgrace to the Iron Maiden.

"Have a good puke?" said my brother Billy. He had the stomach of a whirling dervish.

"I do not like that word," said Mother.

"He's got throw-up on his sleeve," insisted Billy. "It stinks."

"I do not like that word either," said Mother.

At which point Father would reach one arm into the back seat and give Billy a wallop.

"I have to do it again," I would announce.

Even today I do not like riding in a car, would vastly prefer going on foot or taking the train. Actually, I would prefer to stay home while the rest of the family went out for a drive. But they won't let me. So it happened that while out for a Sunday ride not long ago, my second son grew quiet, still, and pale. Then came those words that drove a stake through my heart. "Stop the car." Quickly I pulled off to the side of the road, while the fleet and heartless world whooshed carelessly past. I held the wracked and wretching little boy over what I knew to be the first of countless road-shoulders and ditches all over America. Suddenly I felt a cold chill grip my flesh, and turned to see if someone, something were gaining on me.

LONGFELLOW, VIRGIL, AND ME

To search for one's literary forebears is to hunt a genealogy more intimate by far than the identification of the ancient flesh from which one's mere body has come. It is a quest for saints long since lifted to the glory of Heaven, there to sit at golden tables in the vicinity of God. Within my mind, there are two men to whom I remain belted by filaments of the imagination of such a tensile strength as to have withstood the distraction, the wear and tear of thirty years. These are Longfellow and Virgil (bacia mano). May Heaven with its endless possibilities have brought them to the same table. And there may they wait patiently, patiently for me.

It was early in my schooling that I was required to lisp from memory the poems of Longfellow. So early that I cannot imagine childhood without him. For the children of Troy, New York, in the nineteen thirties, Evangeline, Minne-ha-ha, the village smith, and the skeleton in armor were the great heroic figures of literature. We knew no others. Nor have these poems left me while all else has either dropped like so many stones beneath the black tarn of forgetfulness or blurred into poor approximation or paraphrase. But then who could forget "Grave Alice and laughing Allegra, and Edith with golden hair"?

And, ah, that intrepid youth "who bore 'mid snow and ice,/a banner with the strange device, Excelsior." Where, we died to know, was he going? What implacable fury hounded him up that mountain, as the shades of night were falling fast? What did it mean, Excelsior? Was it the emblem of a promise given? Some cryptic warning? A terrible cri de coeur? It did not matter. The very syllables drove us mad with yearning. We longed to climb with him, side by side, sharing his passion and his agony, to take from his faltering arm that banner, and to wrap ourselves in Excelsior.

More than one voice quavered and broke, more eyes than mine filled with tears as we spoke that heartrending stanza wherein the brawny village smith, sitting in church with his sons, hears his daughter's voice in the choir, and "needs must think of her mother once more, / How in the grave she lies; /And with his hard rough hand he wipes / A tear out of his eyes." Twenty lumps gathered as one in twenty throats as we surrendered our hearts.

Most dreadful of all was the tale of the *Hesperus*, whose skipper had brought his little daughter to keep him company on the voyage. Her eyes were blue "as fairy-flax," her bosom white "as the hawthorn buds that ope in the month of May." With what commingled terror and grief did we see him lifeless and lashed to the helm, all stiff and stark, with his face turned toward the skies. With what sorrow did we later espy the little girl still tied to the drifting mast. "The salt-sea was frozen on her breast." (O bosom white as hawthorn buds.) "The salt tears in her eyes." (Blue as fairy-flax they were.) And her hair "like the brown sea-weed / On the billows fall and rise." Christ save us all, aloud cried we who had seen no waters more turbulent than those of the viscid Hudson, Christ save us all from the reef of Norman's Woe. It is thirty years later; my hair and brain cells fall from my head in a constant dismal rain. Still I murmur a fervent amen.

Most meticulously studied were the teachers. We scrutinized them like scholarly anthropologists, making observations on their habits, mannerisms, clothing, and dispositions. No fanatic rabbinate ruminating on the Talmud raised more convoluted conjecture. Now and then, rumor, like a madness, would sweep the schoolhouse: "Miss Cleary has a boyfriend." "Miss Feerick wears underpants down to her knees." Frissons of excitement infected from one to the other, leaping across the prurient aisles.

There was Gertrude Vaughn, third grade, her face in a permanent open-lipped smile that, by the addition of no more than a single crease, would have become a captured shriek. And Anna Mahoney, kindergarten, whose giant bosom was so tightly impacted upon her chest as to seem one uncleft tumefaction. Her voice was sweet as the billy club that swung at her brother's leg. Her sister Catherine, the principal, wore flat, laced oxfords with flapping external tongues. With each step her head shook from side to side rejecting every possibility.

From across the sea they had come, fierce Celtic maidens, long, long past their prime, and with a collective hunger that made of the potato famine a mere bagatelle. Such were the schoolteachers of Troy, whose indentured mothers had scoured the bathrooms of the middle class to send their girls to Normal School for the certificates that would ensure that *they* would never take lye and plunger to anyone else's toilet. Like a cloud of rare colored moths they had settled on the blackboards and knee-hole desks of Troy. Oh, let me recall them—their hair marcelled into all the waves of the sea, engulfed in opposing clouds of eau-de-cologne which drifted from each room into the corridors where they fought invisible gaseous battles for supremacy; the reckless prints in which they dressed—here lightning streaked across a sleeve, there Chinese poppies pocked a trussed buttocks like some ill-gotten rash, and only lacking was the Spanish Armada in full rout across an abdomen.

Thus, tattooed like Zulus, they patrolled, nodding and smiling to each other above the lines of snot, and the pairs and pairs of famished eyes that stared from one to the other in wildest surmise.

In the classrooms, the Palmer Method of Penmanship vied with Civics like princes of the throne. *Silas Marner* was in dread contention with *Santa Lucia*. But it was Latin that was king of Troy. And if Latin was king, his consort was the relentless, the implacable Ethel Houlihan. No bird of paradise she, but drab as a Quaker, her hair a failed bush, her skin and lips of the same leaden hue, with only the eyes ablaze, febrile. When she was angered her rage became almost tangible: it vaporized from her body; it had a smell, like starch. Howling, writhing, breaking chalk, flinging erasers, she gorged us with Latin. We were geese being primed for paté. Over the ridges of vocabulary she led us, scaling the cruelest cliff of grammar only to find another, steeper just beyond. Past ablatives absolute, ut-clauses of purpose, and grievous gerundives she herded us, pausing only long enough to flagellate the laggards. In *Jason and the Argonauts* she was Medea, crazy, abandoned, slaying her children. In *The Aeneid* she was Dido delivering her seaside lament into the head of a typhoon.

Margaret Byrnes sat three aisles away and one behind me. She was the most woebegone person I have ever seen. Everything she did seemed a last desperate effort after the failure of which there would be nothing to do but an act of self-immolation. She it was who each day bore the first brunt of Ethel Houlihan's morning rage. It was ever thus. The one person least equipped, who pretends no concealment of her ineptitude, is the very one who invites the easiest disaster. Lo, the bursting tigress stalks the herd of impala. Confident, restrained, she seeks out the weakest, the slowest, and *finds* her, frail and fainting in the tall grass. Margaret Byrnes labored half the night to translate fifteen lines of *The Aeneid*. In the morning, pale and trembling, came she to class, and to her Calvary. With what a horrid foreknowledge did she cower at her desk, folding and unfolding a hankie long since damp with perspiration, soon to be sopping with tears. Now and then she would be gripped by a shudder most terrible to behold, would socket up her eyes, staring back into that exhausted brain in which datives and genitives tangled and turned helter-skelter.

Had Margaret Byrnes been stupid, ugly, or mean, perhaps I should not have been moved by her passion. But Margaret Byrnes was beauty itself, a pale lamp, a spike of bright yellow. From out the puffs of her short sleeves, thin arms spoke eloquently all the vulnerabilities that she never once put into words. Nor did she look to her classmates for condolence, but suffered alone all the noble dimensions of her battle. Silent, panicky Joan of Arc being led to the stake with the awful premonition upon her. Each day was her martyrdom reenacted, nails, thorns, cross and all.

"Miss Byrnes," came the dread invocation. "Line 110 . . . Tum Dido . . ."

At the first syllable of her name Margaret Byrnes leaped to her feet as though ejected by some dreadful mechanism beneath her chair. Thus sprung and rigid she waited. Soon she would feel that intimate hot breath in the hollow of her neck, the first pressure of fangs, the spurt and run of her blood.

"Well?" urged Ethel Houlihan.

Almost inaudibly Margaret Byrnes cleared her throat. It was an act so piteous as to cramp the bowels of Caligula. The rest of us were become statuary, awaiting its turn beneath the sledgehammer. We could not, had we dared, bleed for her.

"Then Dido . . . ," began the wretched girl.

"Louder," came the fierce commandment. "And faster."

"Then Dido . . ." Margaret Byrnes' voice faltered again, then rallied.

". . . carried back to her palace the souvenirs of her

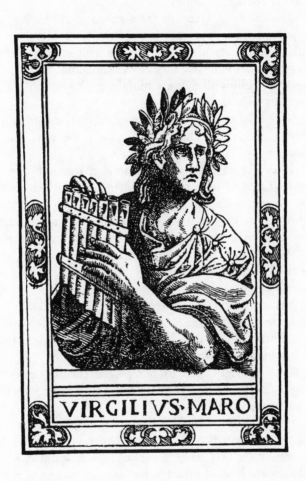

VIRGILIVS·MARO

night in the cave with Aeneas, and fondled them with slowly receding passion."

Not even the freest of translations could have produced a less accurate approximation of the text. The very run of all those consecutive words, each one sprung full-grown from the brow of her fancy, was shocking. What followed was the bellow of a stuck buffalo, a "hoyotoho" to deafen Wotan himself.

"Fool. Moron. Stupid. Yes, you *are* beyond hope, beneath contempt. Once again you have not done your homework."

If ever accusation were falsely charged, this was that time. On and on Ethel Houlihan railed; then, as though overcome with sudden boredom, she tossed the carcass abruptly from her jaws, and ordered the whimpering girl to sit. Which Margaret Byrnes did, folding into the seat.

All through this dark night of the soul, the rest of us waited, like Mary, Queen of Scots, for the thunk of the axe. It came.

"Mister Selzer . . . line 110 . . . Tum Dido."

I rose to my feet.

"Then Dido . . . ," I began, paused, looked up from my book, and continued.

". . . carried back to her palace the souvenirs of her night in the cave with Aeneas, and fondled them with slowly receding passion."

I too had not recited Virgil, nor anything remotely like it, but the words of Margaret Byrnes verbatim. A terrible silence such as I have never known descended upon the classroom. It was as though we were in fact to be present at a beheading.

"What?" whispered Ethel Houlihan, and the wind from that *wh* would have blown Aeneas all the way from Carthage to Italy. Once again the storm rose; the sky turned black; gigantic waves slid beneath my little boat. I yawed; I spun; I lashed myself to the mast, and turned my salt-streaked face heavenward; like the skipper of the *Hesperus*, I made ready to die.

"Answer me, Selzer." She had dropped the mister. It would not go well with me.

"Or it will not go well with you."

But the answer was unspeakable. I had not *planned* to recite the words of Margaret Byrnes, did not know that I would until I had done it. *Now* I know that it was because they were beautiful and true. They were the words of one who knew the human heart better than Longfellow, better than Virgil, better by far than Christiaan Barnard. Virgil *should* have written them.

At the exact moment that Margaret Byrnes uttered them, I fell recklessly in love with her. Those words were her glove; mine, a vow of fealty, my pledge. In that careening sea, I searched and found her face, and to my everlasting glory, flashed her a smile of such heartbreaking courage as to qualify me for first mate aboard the *Golden Hind*.

What happened next remains one of the half-dozen most important events of my life—for back to me from Margaret Byrnes came slowly, shyly, but undeniably *there*, the pale and lovely reflection of my own smile. Here was no mere gesture of gratitude, but an exchange of the heart. Between those two smiles (O measure them in quanta, in light-years) a rainbow arced; there was sealed a covenant, a secret troth plighted. In that moment Margaret Byrnes and I had won no mere present and future, but a past—a past that indeed one day it would be pleasing to remember.

JACOB STREET

Of one thing I am convinced—that there are on the earth certain special places laden with possibility, where anything can happen, magic, supernal, where the laws of matter and electricity suspend their governance, and where a strange and sacred vacancy hovers just above the surface, across which no insect flits, no shadow of man is cast.

Such are the fens of Ireland where, I am told, one can hear the fairies sing, and the meadows in Spain where on certain saintly evenings one can catch the pearly flashings of angels alighting from columns of air. Here are manna and sweet dew upon the ground, and the atmosphere prickles with little stings of delight. These are the interfaces between heaven and earth, the entryways to Paradise.

I know of one such place. It is called Jacob Street. Within its six blocks lived the Armenians of Troy. Fate must have worn her most enigmatic smile when she stood atop the highest hills of Troy and unrolled Jacob Street down to the banks of the Hudson River like an exquisite Oriental carpet, and declared it hallowed ground. Narrow and steep is Jacob Street. It is a ladder that asks a dangerous shift in the center of gravity of him who would climb it. One's chin hangs forward and low like a lantern searching the ground. Long ago Jacob Street had given up all pretensions to modernity and had accepted the slow and gentle desuetude that prevailed when, as a boy, I stood at its foot and gazed up into the crumble of stoops, the mad crookedness of the houses with their lynx-eyed windows.

To ascend into Jacob Street was to enter an ancient rocky land. Moab, perhaps. One's very eyes changed color. The cobblestones were broken and uneven, the sidewalks cracked so that weeds burst in profusion through the fissures. On either side, the houses abutted each other with no space between save occasional narrow alleyways guarded by filigreed wooden gates. Behind these gates hideous mongrels moaned. From these alleys emanated a smell of garlic and roses.

"Keep away from Jacob Street," my mother had said. "Stay where you belong."

But she had not counted on magic. One evening I stood at the foot of the hill and half-heard, half-palpated the sound of music. Strings stretched across ancient oiled wood were being plucked; there was the floating moan of a woman's voice, singing, and a strange thump that came unexpectedly as though a muscle set deep beneath the ground were contracting slowly, erratically. Of course, I went to Jacob Street. And peered at last through a wooden grille, down a dark alley between two houses into a backyard. It was like looking through a telescope at some just-discovered land. At one end of the yard a table had been set up, covered with a white cloth. On it were platters of baklava and meat rolled in cabbage and bottles of colorless brandy. There was the smell of clove and cinnamon. In the center of the yard, a young man in shirtsleeves was dancing, swinging from the handkerchief of another man, turning, stamping, flicking his hips like a whip. And all about, women stood, clapping out the rhythm, their eyes gone muzzy with longing. I was to come back here the next evening, and the one after that.

Deep in the casbah of Jacob Street dwelt Armine der

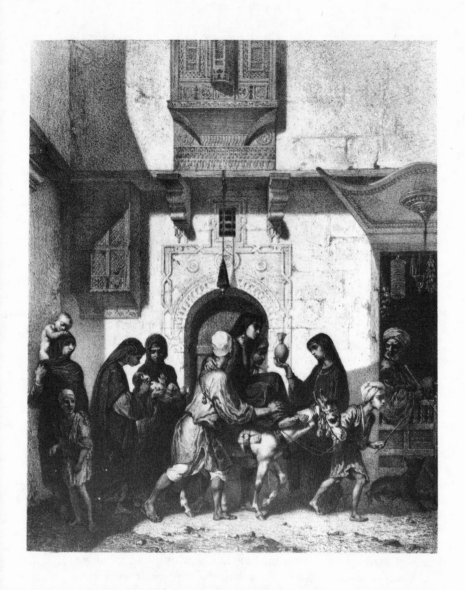

Arakelian. I first saw her sitting on a stoop in what I have ever since thought of as the Persian position. The sole of her right foot was placed against the inner aspect of her left thigh. Her left leg lay gently flexed before her. One hand rested in her lap like a white waterbird. No stance or posture has invited me so. Black of hair was Armine, and with the wispy sideburns with which Mediterranean women are early decorated. Her breasts were twin mythologies—Persian and Arabic—and her nose was a downcurved arch of lewd cartilage. Once having caught sight of that pink tongue furling between her teeth, I was ready to die for her. It was for Armine that I wrote my first poem. I recall only that it rhymed dwarf with wharf.

I do not know how it came to be that Armine der Arakelian and I found ourselves one dusk standing together in the very center of a ten-by-twelve antique Baluchistan rug with a central medallion and a three-layered border of cypress trees and pomegranates. I suppose that a glance of a certain type would have been exchanged, followed by a hush in which could be heard the music of the spheres. Might she then have given me a sign? A small touch, perhaps, that brushed my finest sense hairs?

Probably, she rose slowly, turned into the alley, and mounted the narrow back stairs without looking to see whether I followed. No need. She could have been certain of that. Small fires would have trailed my hooves. That we stood together on the rug, I know; that we faced each other, that I saw again that terrible pink tongue in the center of her face, as challenging as the flag of a mysterious adversary—all this I remember. Of the rest, of what followed, I know only as a man remembers delirium. Something eludes me—I think it is the truth. Yet who is to say that dream is less than memory? Are not both subject to the laws of probability?

Upstairs in the parlor, only the Armenian moon was at home. Its white dust lay thick upon the walls and ceiling.

All at once there was an unsteadiness at my feet, a shifting of my balance. I looked down to see a movement in the rug, as of water running over mosaic tiles, water in which my feet had sunk. In a moment my knees were submerged. I could not have extricated myself had I wished to. A delicious weightiness overtook me. My very organs seemed to have been rearranged. Even my vision was in transition. Now the rug had risen into twin rolling mounds on either side of us, Armine and me, and was flowing down into a central vortex. Together we lay backward upon it and sank into the cream of the carpet. And all the while, light and air flowed through me, running upon my lips and eyes.

When I opened my eyes, I was aware of the musty smell of the rug.

"You'd better go," said Armine. The buttons of my shirt had turned to mucilage.

I closed the door to the back stairs, and started down. When I looked back, Armine had vanished. And try as I might to cling to the details of that evening, with each step downward, they slipped one after the other through the net of memory, until they were as far away and irretrievable as the stars. As I took the last of those steps, I had forgotten all and had left only what I have written here.

But of such delight one somehow needs proof. Why did not a fountain spring from that site to burble forever down the hills of Troy? Were white-winged Pegasus ever to touch alabaster hoof to earth once more, it should have been to this place, to mark it forever.

It is so many years later, so far from Troy. On the floor of my study, where I sit scribbling these words, there is an Oriental rug. Baluchistan, I think. Often and again I turn to gaze at it. Sometimes I see the colors swirl, the patterns blend. There is a movement like water running over mosaic tiles. If I stare long enough, twin mounds appear. There is a rolling . . .

BIRDWATCHING

One would think it no disgrace to lack excellence in bird-watching. But there are those in every pursuit who lie in wait to heap shame upon ridicule. It was ever thus, and no different among the "gentle" spies on earth's aviary. Of course, great expectations, even as Charles Dickens has taught, are invariably unfulfilled, and what look, at first glance, like innocent flowers are the serpents underneath.

Can a person who watches birds be all bad? Yes, Yes, I tell you yes. It is the birdwatcher who, with his incessant vying, desecrates the forests and seacoasts, the cliffs and bogs of our land. You have not met perfect cruelty until you have spent an entire day crouching among thorns, smorgasbord for the entire insect kingdom, your neck become a solid column of pain from gazing upward through impacted masses of foliage at what you thought was something flitting (a bird) but which turns out to be something rustling (a leaf). And all for a glimpse of a single rose-breasted grosbeak. At last, at last it is evening. You concede defeat and hie homeward your humid hurting feet. But what is this? Rounding a bend in the path you come upon a lone figure writing furiously in a notebook. The slouch, the suggestion of the ramshackle, the touch of decrepitude, and the necklace of field glasses identify him as a bird-watcher.

On guard! Expect no affable camaraderie, no gripping of arms, no warm effusion. You pause to observe him from a distance, every wary nerve come suddenly alive. You study him through your glasses. A little smile plays about his mouth, beneath which squats a beard so like the nest of the Baltimore Oriole as to set you peering therein for eggs. Now and then he interrupts his writing to pop an unidentified seed into his mouth with a smug little bob of his head. With mounting discomfort you notice that he is wearing a black hat and an orange shirt. He is making out his *List*.

A quick look at your own confirms the sad account: a fish crow, two robins, and one pigeon alone and palely loitering. Be still, heart. You have not yet been seen. You are a deer, grass at lip, one leg aloft and poised for flight, listening to the distant rumble of thunder. . . . Quickly. Cast about for an alternate path by which one might avoid the confrontation. There is none. Your eye falls upon a fist-sized rock at your feet. You stoop to pick it up.

"Good evening," he says. It is too late. The rock falls from your fingers with a dispirited thud. And the play begins. For him, *H.M.S. Pinafore;* for you *Götterdämmerung.*

"Did you see the hooded warblers?" He pricks with the kind of studied nonchalance that is apter in the cloakrooms of the Senate than on the footpaths of Acadia.

"Why, no. I didn't." You are perspiring, and feel a terrible itch in your palm. You gauge the distance between yourself and the rock.

"How about the little green heron?" He is blooded now, and thrusting home.

"Missed that one too. Darn." You are all sheepishness, and toe-scraping bumbler.

"Nice old Northern wood thrush, wasn't it?" He is arch as a diplomat.

"Oh, dear." He turns to scribble in his pad. "I almost forgot the rose-breasted grosbeak."

Oh, a hit! A palpable hit! And you are stung. *Your* bird. *Your* rose-breasted grosbeak. Oh, perverse bird, to have hidden from view only to hawk thy wares before this descendant of the Marquis de Sade. May you become extinct for that, grosbeak. I am diminished; mine enemy thrives; he waxes great.

You leap upon him, seize the straps of his field glasses, and twist them slowly, slowly in the wind, until his face grows empurpled as any martin or finch. Pulling the hideous head close, you hiss between grinding teeth, "Assassin! Criminal! Do you know that I am partially color-blind? That blue and gray and green and brown are all the same to me? That I am trying to overcome it?" You can feel your lower lip trembling, as the passion rises.

"Now did *you* see the archeopteryx down the road? The pair of nesting pterodactyls?" Even as you thrust the carcass from you, a mockingbird pumps music from his throat. It is your best sighting of the day.

Among the things that birdwatching is more fun than is jogging, which is the sweaty, self-righteous business of pious accountants and suchlike, all with their gaze fixed firmly on longevity, as opposed to eternity, which is what birdwatching is all about. Personally, I regard jogging, cold showers, and flagellation with whips as perversions, and not the interesting kind. I fully expect a college of High Cardiologists to announce one day that, heh, heh, jogging is, after all, injurious to your health.

When a jogger passes a birdwatcher on a path in the park, there is, if not fisticuffs, electricity. I would prefer the former, and one day, I swear it, I shall leap from my painful blind, seize the fool, and *together* we shall scare the birds away.

That I am still numbered among the Birdwatchers of

America is due to no persistent craving for fellowship or lusting after lists. What is it, then, this need that is no less than an obsession? Is it that, short of flying, there is watching birds fly? Is it that, songless, I crave the flute of the wood thrush? Lacking plumage, I revel in tanagers? I understand you, Leda. You and your private swantics. I too would soar, sing, display, dine and mate with birds. They are the imagination concretized. They are a distraction from death. I watch the birds. It is myself that I see.

Still it is the little meannesses that beckon as well as the beauties, the carbuncles among the rubies. Thus the butchery of the loggerhead shrike which, having caught a mouse by the tail, flies it swinging into a thorn bush to impale it. It is easier to feast upon skewered meat. The villainy of the oxpecker is more cunning, Watergatian. His name is misleading. He does not look at all like that. He is, rather, a nondescript fellow who uses his bill as a scissors to slice ticks from the hides of cattle. It is not, however, the flesh of the tick for which it hungers, but the blood of the ox with which the insect is engorged. Like a politician who professes to do good for the body politic, the oxpecker slyly feeds upon the great beast's blood in parasitism most treacherous. The cedar waxwing feeds upon chokecherries with a hunger so reckless that he does not stop until he is filled to the very tip of his bill. Nor can he close it, and the last cherry falls from the tip to the ground despite that he holds it aloft to retain it. He tries to fly, but cannot. He is too heavy. Soon the chokecherries ferment, and the delirious waxwing flops about, tipping his wings this way and that. All about the bush he staggers, a drunk leaving a saloon at closing time.

One ought to listen and respond to the little warnings of what I persist, against all reason, in believing to be a benevolent nature. In retrospect I should have known when I learned that the Latin name for the robin is *Turdus migratorius*. The decline and fall of illusion was as abrupt as that

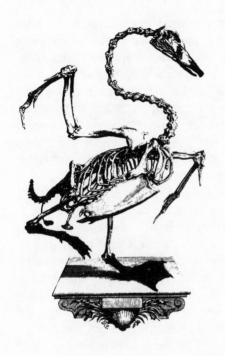

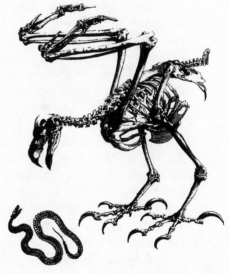

of Icarus when his own feathered glory turned runny on his shoulders. Never again was I to see a robin as anything else but flying *rejectimenta*. Farewell to Robin Redbreast, harbinger of spring. Now I turn my gaze lawnwise to see robins mincing arrogantly on the grass, and it is as though a dog had been very naughty thereupon. But then watch an egret unship his oars and row away, solve the message of clawtracks on a beach, hear pigeons applauding themselves to your windowsill, or the distant drumming of a partridge, and wonder.

In *The New York Times* one read that in certain parts of South Africa ostriches are being used to herd sheep. A dark and dangerous precedent. It is no less than the introduction of a power structure into the world of the beasts. Thus will their corruption be assured. Birdwatcher though I am, I must confess that in such an adversary relationship my sympathies lie with the sheep. No more do the plumes of the ostrich ravish my vision. I see only the bald neck, the horrid pink head, those sledgehammer feet. Consider the scene. Behold the hired ostrich, his arrogant plumage astir with easy rage, his bullet head rocking with military precision atop the rubbery neck. With three giant strides he catches the luckless laggard lamb and *whomp, bam*, right into eternity. What can you expect from a stupid creature that, bald as its egg, wears its colors on its backside? And whither? one might well ask. Whither the ostrich? Is it lebensraum next? A wehrmacht? Is there a herrenvolk abuilding? From sheep to goats, then on to cattle until all the beasts of the field are ringed and cordoned? It is but a short leap thence to human beings—political prisoners, slanderers of the establishment, users of marijuana and other pests. See men such as these set out in meadows, encircled by angry strutting ostriches so testy that a sneeze would be interpreted by them as a revolutionary act and altogether deserving of a severe stomping.

Students of the psyche would do well to watch birds. I

think of the nonbreeding swift who, at the signal of twilight, ascends in slowly mounting circles to great invisible heights. All the night long it floats in delirious arcs above the clouds. Nor does it feed up there nor do anything but join with the elements in galactic ecstasy. Or the Andean hummingbird which, when touched or threatened, falls into a state of torpor so profound as to mimic death. The very functions of its body are willed to a standstill. These two, at least, have quite simply gotten off the treadmill.

In the New Haven, Connecticut, telephone book, on page 99, entitled DAN–DAV, there is a little square space in the very center of the page. It contains this information:

DARK ENTRY . . . near Cornwall Bridge, a mysterious area, formerly known as Owlsbury, where a number of people who attempted to make their homes all lost their sanity. In 1854 there were four houses hidden among the dense thickets, but by 1871 there were none. Many great horned owls now inhabit the area.

Something sinister is going on, and we are drawn to it as Pandora to her box, as Orpheus to Hades. It is an ancient allure, fetid and swampy. Upon what did those early settlers so irresistibly gaze, the sight of which drove them mad? Was it some birdish deviltry set them giggling in those dense thickets? Laid them frothing? Into what concealment went those four little houses, whisked whole or crumbled into smoke? And more, what became of the maniacs themselves? Were they beaked and clawed by ravenous owls, or *are* they the owls, become so by some black and feathered transubstantiation, doomed to hoot forever like souls in torment? Now I go to Dark Entry and listen to the owls screeching through the trees, and I tremble, and feel a little madness of my own.

PICTURE CREDITS

The author and publisher wish to thank the following for kind permission to reproduce the material listed below:

YALE MEDICAL LIBRARY:

I am delighted to acknowledge the assistance of Susan Klein and Ferenc Gyorgyey of the Yale Medical Historical Library in the location and selection of illustrative material. My thanks also to Beverly Pope and Roy Carlson.

ABOUT THE AUTHOR

Richard Selzer was for many years a surgeon practicing in New Haven, Connecticut, where he was also on the faculty of the Yale School of Medicine. He was born in 1928 in Troy, New York, was graduated from Union College and Albany Medical College, and from the Surgical Training Program of Yale University.

In 1975 he won the National Magazine Award for his essays on medicine.

Dr. Selzer has retired from medical practice and from teaching to pursue writing full-time.

He lives with his wife in New Haven.